EQUINE FITNESS

EQUINE FITNESS

The Care and Training of the Athletic Horse

Dr. D H Snow and
C J Vogel

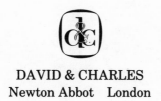

DAVID & CHARLES
Newton Abbot   London

British Library Cataloguing in Publication Data

Snow, David
    Equine Fitness: The Care and Training of the Athletic Horse
    1. Horses——Training
    I. Title II. Vogel, Colin
    636.1'083   SF287

    ISBN 0-7153-8732-2

Typeset by ABM Typographics Limited, Hull
and printed in Great Britain
by Redwood Burn Limited, Trowbridge, Wilts
for David & Charles Publishers plc
Brunel House   Newton Abbot   Devon

Contents

List of Illustrations

Line Drawings

Plates

This book is dedicated to the equine athletes of the past, in the hope that it will enable the horse owners to train more wisely the equine athletes of the future and thus continue to bring pleasure to millions of participants and observers.

Preface

by HRH The Princess Anne

Equestrian sports depend on the welfare of the horse for its success – from racing to Pony Club Games – but not all human participants in equestrian sports i.e. trainers and riders – understand the demands which they make on their horses. Competition is hotter than ever – due largely to sheer weight of numbers and there being many more opportunities to compete. The trainer/rider needs help to achieve the correct level of equine fitness which is not only important for achieving success, but in avoiding unnecessary suffering and prolonging the active life of our equine partners.

This book goes back to some basic biological and scientific facts and through collaboration between an active research worker and a practising veterinary surgeon, there is here a book where the interested lay person can read, with a greater chance of understanding, what modern science is beginning to learn about the athletic horse. A number of old ideas are more than questioned but it does no harm to have pet ideas challenged – equally, it's worth the scientists remembering that the horse is not going to read this book and may well not be so impressed with their arguments!

Horses need to be fit in body and mind – like any athlete – in order to produce their best and when more questions are being asked about the safety of equestrian sports, their preparation becomes even more crucial. I hope that 'Equine Fitness' will help us all to improve the standards of fitness, the standard of competition and quite possibly the success that we can achieve with our remarkable equine partners.

Anne

Introduction

During the past thirty-five years or so there has been a tremendous explosion of interest in the horse all over the world. To some extent, this may have been due to a need to retain some contact with the 'living world' at a time when our lives have become more and more mechanised. There has also been a gradual increase in the amount of leisure time which we all enjoy. Hand in hand with this growing interest has come an increase in the number of competitions open to the horse and rider. In 1985 the horse population in the USA was estimated to be 8,519,000 with by far the largest number of horses being used for pleasure, exhibition or competition purposes.

Horses have probably been raced by their owners for as long as they have been ridden. There is an engraving from the Dordogne of a horse with a halter which is thought to be ten thousand years old, and horses were certainly being ridden in the area known as Persia and Mesopotamia five thousand years ago. Newmarket is sometimes called the home of racing because of its long history of organised race-meetings which date back to the reign of King Charles I. Of course, in those days training and feeding methods were very different from those of today. In 1599, for instance, it is recorded that racehorses were fed bread. 'Goode bigge white' loaves for this purpose cost 1d.

Racing is still as popular as ever throughout the world, with Thoroughbred horses being raced in countries such as Malaysia and Hong Kong, where the breed is a modern introduction, and both Standardbred and Quarterhorse racing very much on the up-swing. Nevertheless, the real explosion of interest has been in the so-called competition world. Although racing remains the 'sport of kings', a new world has opened up for the less well off who have to combine the roles of owner, groom, rider, and competitions secretary.

This book aims to explain how the horse functions as an athlete. Although scientific research has lagged behind the horse-owning public's desire to know why some horses perform better than others, and why some people can train a horse more successfully than others, a great deal of progress is now being made. Wherever possible, the very latest scientific findings have been incorporated into the text. Some of them are controversial, some may upset traditionalists, but all have the great virtue of being demonstrated scientifically. The authors do not claim that everyone who reads this book will be able to train a Derby winner, or win an Olympic gold medal at showjumping, but they should be able to understand better what they are doing to their horse during the training process.

The book is written for those interested in gaining an insight into how their horses function, so that they can develop their personal training methods in a rational way which is based on scientific fact rather than myth. We might make an analogy to a car. One can drive a car without understanding its intricacies, but to obtain optimum performance from it, one will need to understand some of its workings. One might carry the analogy further, and liken the chassis of the car to the skeleton of the horse. The engine is then equivalent to the muscles of the horse, and in the same way that the carburettor, radiator and exhaust help the engine, so do the horse's lungs, heart, kidneys, etc back up the muscles. There is, however, a very big difference between a car and a horse. Although they both have a 'driver', the horse also has a brain of its own which we ignore at our peril. The aim of the horse-rider or trainer must be to combine their knowledge with the inherent ability of the horse and thus to achieve more than would otherwise have been possible.

By explaining how the athletic horse functions, we will also hopefully counteract some of the ignorance which has developed as modern society has grown away from the animal-based culture which used to provide good examples for people to follow. The novice horse owner is subjected to a barrage of advertising from feed-supplement manufacturers, etc. Not everything which is presented in advertisements as modern science has any true scientific basis at all. It is certainly possible to improve the economics of keeping an athletic horse by studying what is scientifically necessary in the fields of nutrition, etc. It is also important that we do not achieve any improvements in performance at the horse's expense. So much of modern veterinary research in the field of exercise physiology is aimed at reducing still further any distress which we might inadvertently cause our horses during normal equine activities. In this respect, we should point out that it is the authors' view that drugs are for temporary use to cure specific veterinary conditions rather than for the masking of problems which would otherwise limit success in athletic competitions.

How the modern athletic horse has evolved
The different fields of equine endeavour make varying demands on the horse. When horses are sprinting over short distances, such as the ¼ mile

(400m) covered by the aptly named Quarterhorses, or the 5 and 6 fur-longs (1,000 and 1,200m) of conventional flat-race sprints, the horse requires the ability to obtain an enormous amount of energy very quickly in order to keep its legs moving at full speed. A horse racing over middle distances of between 1 and 2 miles (1,600 and 3,200m), on the other hand, will not need its energy quite so quickly but requires the ability to sustain high-power output for longer periods. Steeplechasing requires even more stamina, but the speed of the race will be slower still, and the rhythm of the horse is continually being broken by the need to jump.

The dressage horse may never need to gallop at all during either training or competition, but its muscles must be extremely supple and its gait perfectly even. Showjumping is, perhaps, the least demanding discipline of all as regards fitness. The horses are in the showjumping ring only for a couple of minutes, during which they are not moving at any great speed and will never be trotting in a straight line long enough for anyone to notice any minor stiffness. Horse-trials enthusiasts con-sider that their sport is the most complete test of a horse's all-round ability and fitness because the cross-country phase requires both speed and endurance to complement the dressage and showjumping phases. In three-day events, the horses are rested overnight between the cross-country and showjumping phases, but must pass a veterinary inspection before showjumping. Muscles have to be working very efficiently indeed if they are not to show signs of stiffness (which may be synonymous with a certain degree of muscle pain) on that third morning. It would be in-teresting to go around a large number of racehorses on the morning after a race and trot them out to see whether they are sound or not.

Although various kinds of equine competition require stamina, the long-distance riding competition can be considered the true endurance test and places a specialised demand on the horse. Energy is required at a steady level which must be maintained for many hours. Owing to the length of the competition, the horse must dispose of the waste products of its energy production as it goes along; it cannot do so at its leisure afterwards. Sweating and temperature control become vitally important in this situation.

It would not be possible for any one horse to excel in all these different fields of equine competition. We live in the age of the specialist, and the horse breeds are no exception. There have probably always been at least three types of horse, even in prehistoric times before the horse was domesticated, some four thousand years ago.

The first of these ancient types of horse was the horse which lived on the steppes. We still have a living example of this type in the Przewalski horse which was discovered on the Mongolian steppes by Colonel N. Przewalski in 1881 and is still preserved in zoos. The second basic horse type inhabited the forests. They were comparatively heavy and slow moving. Their modern descendants are the heavy horse breeds and ponies. They are often referred to as the 'cold-blooded' breeds. Most modern 'warm-blooded' horses have evolved from the horses which inhabited the plateau lands. They are thought to have been the lightest of the three types, with a finer build than the others. Even in those prehistoric times the limbs and feet of the different horse types had different characteristics. The soup-plate like hooves of our Draught Horses were already present in the horses of the forests, for instance, while the other types had much finer limbs and feet suitable for travelling at faster speeds, thus enabling them to escape the predators in these regions.

The oldest breed of domesticated horse is the Arab. There is certainly evidence that the Arab existed about 2000BC, and an eighth-century historian known as El Kelbi recorded pedigrees reaching back to the time of Bax, a great-great-great-grandson of Noah. If Solomon was, as has been suggested, the greatest horse dealer of all time by virtue of his 1,200 saddle horses and 40,000 chariot horses, the present interest shown by middle-eastern families has been almost as revolutionary in its effect on the bloodstock markets.

Encouraged by Mohammed to attain paradise by paying particular attention to the care of the horse, the Arabs developed a breed of horse renowned both for its strength and its beauty. It is interesting to speculate whether the *mitbah* of the Arab, the curved arch of the head and neck which is so different from the sharp angle so beloved by modern dressage enthusiasts, has contributed to the breed's stamina by ensuring an unobstructed airway.

The modern Thoroughbred owes a great deal to the Arab. Cross-bred horses were used by the English nobility for racing from the Middle Ages, and Arab blood was almost certainly being continually mixed in with the native blood. Three Arab stallions in particular shaped the Thoroughbred because all present members of the breed can trace back to them on the male side. The first of these imports was the Byerley Turk, who founded the Herod line. The Godolphin Arabian was imported in 1728, and was responsible for the Matchem line. The last of these three founder stallions was the Darley Arabian, who sired Flying Childers and Eclipse and who retired from the racecourse unbeaten in 1760.

The first General Stud Book was published by Weatherby's in 1791 and the same firm are still responsible for keeping records of all Thoroughbreds in the United Kingdom and Eire. Nowadays, enormous sums of money are paid at public auction for Thoroughbred yearlings which are far too young to give much idea about their future physical build but which are bred out of fashionable bloodstock lines. The racing form book shows us that there are probably as many well-bred horses which do not come up to expectations as there are fashionable purchases who strike gold for their owners. Proven performance is the only true guide to a racehorse's value to the breed as a whole because that performance demonstrates that the horse has the physical structure (in conformation and in microscopic cellular anatomy) to succeed. The hunt is, however, very much on to perfect scientific means of predicting racehorse performance, and some of these techniques will be discussed later.

The early Thoroughbreds were called on to race over a variety of distances, with the heats being over 3 or 4 miles (4,800 and 6,400m). In the nineteenth century, there was a reduction in the distances, and most of the races were over a mile (1,600m) or more. This is still reflected by the fact that all the English Classic races (the 1,000 Guineas, the 2,000 Guineas, the Derby, the Oaks, and the St Leger) are middle-distance races rather than sprints. It has only been in comparatively recent years that shorter distances have become more popular, and the fashion for racing two-year-olds hard rather than waiting for them to mature has had some influence on this. The trend to race two-year-olds has been especially marked in the USA. It may well be that racing at such an early age is detrimental to the long-term interests of the horses because of the extreme forces which are placed on immature bones. Interestingly, in Hong Kong, where all the racehorses are purchased from other countries, horses are barred from running until they are three years old. The desire of the betting public for a quick result has been another factor in promoting shorter races. The really famous household names in a Thoroughbred's pedigree will almost certainly be these middle-distance horses, which is a point to bear in mind when buying a Thoroughbred for a purpose other than racing, eg eventing.

The American Quarterhorse, on the other hand, evolved solely to race over one specific distance, 1/4 mile (400m), although nowadays they do race over other distances as well. It is said that the early settlers in Virginia and the Carolinas used to race their fastest horses down the main streets on Sunday afternoons. As these streets were rarely more than 1/4 mile (400m) long, the horses became named after the distance of the race. Originally, of course, the breed were primarily cattle horses, noted for their quick turning ability when roping steers as well as their speed. Today, however, there are essentially two types of Quarterhorse: the traditional animal which competes in various events to test both agility and speed, and the racing Quarterhorse. The latter is often at least three-quarters Thoroughbred, being selected from the tested sprinters of that breed. Being bred for a specialised purpose, it has a rather specialised conformation. The back is relatively short, but the hind-quarters are very strong and well-developed in order to enable the horse to get off to a flying start. When looked at from behind, the quarters are even wider at the stifles than they are at the hips. A good Quarterhorse can cover ¼ mile (400m) in as little as twenty seconds, but despite this burst of speed it would be no match against a Thoroughbred at 1 mile (1,600m) or even 6 furlongs (1,200m). The Quarterhorse's other claim to fame is that it is the most numerous breed in the world, thanks to its enormous popularity in the USA.

Like the Quarterhorse, the American Standardbred has Thorough-bred ancestors. When the American Trotting Register was started in 1871, all horses had to be able to trot or pace a mile (1,600m) in a stan-dard time. The original standards were 2 minutes 30 seconds at the trot, and 2 minutes 25 seconds at the pace. The true 'pace', incidentally, is a gait where both the front and hind feet on one side strike the ground to-gether, followed by the front and hind feet of the other side. In conforma-tion, the Standardbred is heavier boned than the Thoroughbred, with more marked sloping of the quarters. The quarters themselves are very well developed, rather like those of the Quarterhorse. The nostrils should be capable of immense flaring, which is said to help oxygen in-take when the horse is travelling at speed.

Although trotting has never rivalled flat-racing and National Hunt racing in popularity in the UK, this is not the case in other parts of the world. In northern Europe, trotting is far and away the most popular kind of horse racing, and in the USA there are around eight hundred trotting tracks. The incidence of various types of lameness in trotters can vary considerably from those found in Thoroughbred racehorses, and this can lead to some confusion when veterinary surgeons from differ-ent parts of the world are discussing the relative importance of such disorders.

By and large, horse racing in its varied forms tends to be closely allied to pure bred horses of one breed or another. It might even be a condition imposed by the ruling body of the sport that only horses registered in a particular stud book may take part, as is the case with the Jockey Club in the UK which requires all horses racing on the flat under their juris-diction to be registered in the Thoroughbred stud book kept by Messrs Weatherby (who act as the Jockey Club's agent). Competition horses, on the other hand, tend to be drawn from a much wider range of breeds and cross-breeds. Some countries have made great strides in recording the breeding of these pleasure horses and promoting their sale on an international basis. Germany, for example, has been so successful in this sphere that many of the leading showjumpers of the world are pure- or part-bred Hanoverians.

Despite the variety of activities which are undertaken in the competitive horse world, training methods have become rather stereotyped. Owners of showjumpers and eventers, for instance, have tended to base their general fitness training on the methods which have evolved in large Thoroughbred racing establishments. This involves trotting and slow canter work every day, with a fast gallop once or twice a week. In recent years, however, a new school of thought has gained some popularity in the eventing world. This uses interval training, the theory of which is that the horses must walk and trot every day. Then, about every third day, they undergo 'interval training' which involves a variable number of alternating periods of cantering and trotting. The trotting periods are adjusted in length to allow the horse's heart rate to slow down to a standard exercising level before the horse does another piece of faster work. By reducing the amount of fast work done at any one stretch, it is hoped to avoid the risk of excessive strain being placed on fatigued muscles, etc. Although it might be claimed that the standard training methods have stood the test of time, it might also be said that the fact that race times have remained relatively static over the past years (in contrast to the situation in human athletics where records are broken almost every week) is due to a failure on the part of the equine world to use the knowledge we are beginning to acquire in equine exercise physiology. If we are to obtain the maximum benefit from this knowledge, we must first go back to the basics of the horse's anatomy.

1 · Anatomy for Performance

Most readers will be familiar with the horse's skeleton, even if they could not give a name to any of the bones (Fig 1). The skeleton cannot move the horse forward one inch without its very complicated system of muscles. All horses, no matter what their breed, size, or their function, have the same arrangement of muscles. With specialisation, however, certain muscles may be better developed in particular horses. If the skin of a horse were to be removed, the superficial muscles would become visible (Fig 2). Although there are other, deeper, muscles, it is the superficial muscles which are also the main muscles of movement and so the muscles which interest us most in the athletic horse.

The head and neck
When considering the muscles of movement, we must start with the muscles which support the head. The horse's head weighs a consider-able amount, and because it is positioned at the end of a long lever (the neck), it requires relatively powerful muscles to support it. The muscles are helped by a large sheet of elastic tissue called the ligamentum nuchae. This stretches from the skull back to the withers, and connects with all the vertebrae in the neck. It acts as an anchorage point in the midline of the neck onto which the muscles can attach. The splenius muscle, for instance, attaches to the ligamentum nuchae and controls the movement of the head either up and down or from side to side.

It is a general principle with muscles that every muscle has an oppos-ing partner which acts in the opposite direction. If one thinks in terms of the muscles running along the top two-thirds of the neck as supporting the spine, the muscles along the bottom third of the neck must work in unison with them, otherwise the horse's head would spend most of its time up in the air. This is because muscles use energy to contract; they do not have an actual mechanism to stretch themselves again. In the case of the head carriage, if the splenius muscle contracts, it lifts the head up. With time and the effect of the head's weight, the head would drop down when the splenius stopped contracting but this would not be a quick and controlled movement. In any case, when the head did drop down it would drop right down to the ground. So there has to be a com-

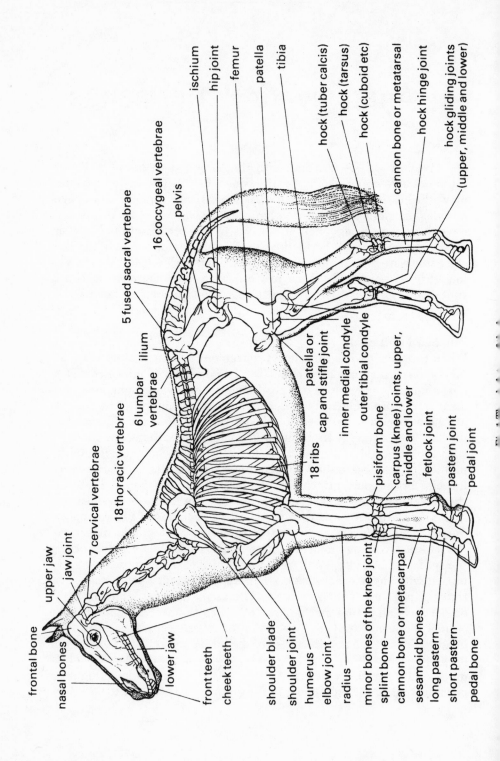

frontal bone
nasal bones
upper jaw
jaw joint
7 cervical vertebrae
18 thoracic vertebrae
lower jaw
front teeth
cheek teeth
shoulder blade
shoulder joint
humerus
elbow joint
radius
minor bones of the knee joint
splint bone
cannon bone or metacarpal
sesamoid bones
long pastern
short pastern
pedal bone

6 lumbar vertebrae
ilium
5 fused sacral vertebrae
16 coccygeal vertebrae
pelvis

ischium
hip joint
femur
patella
tibia
hock (tuber calcis)
hock (tarsus)
hock (cuboid etc)
cannon bone or metatarsal
hock hinge joint
hock gliding joints (upper, middle and lower)

18 ribs
patella or cap and stifle joint
inner medial condyle
outer tibial condyle
pisiform bone
carpus (knee) joints, upper, middle and lower
fetlock joint
pastern joint
pedal joint

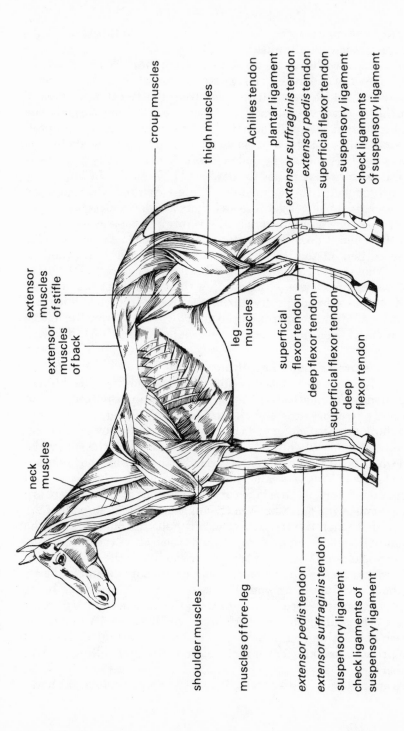

neck
muscles

extensor
muscles
of stifle

extensor
muscles
of back

croup muscles

thigh muscles

Achilles tendon

plantar ligament

extensor suffraginis tendon

extensor pedis tendon

superficial flexor tendon

suspensory ligament

check ligaments
of suspensory ligament

leg
muscles

superficial
flexor tendon

deep flexor tendon

superficial flexor tendon

deep
flexor tendon

shoulder muscles

muscles of fore-leg

extensor pedis tendon

extensor suffraginis tendon

suspensory ligament

check ligaments of
suspensory ligament

Fig 2 The muscles of the horse

plementary system acting in the opposite direction, in this case, for instance, the sterno-cephalic muscle.

Not all of the muscles along the bottom part of the neck are concerned with movement of the neck itself. There is a muscle called the sterno-thyro-hyoideus which runs all the way from the sternum, or breast-bone, to the larynx or voice-box. The importance of this muscle and some of its fellows is that they pull down the larynx to enable the horse to swallow. Occasionally, you get a horse which is said to swallow its tongue when it is hard pressed at the end of a race. What actually happens is that these muscles have pulled too hard, and have pulled the larynx out of its 'buttonhole' in the soft palate. The air coming in through the horse's nose can no longer get into its larynx and down to its lungs, and the horse slows down rapidly and makes a gurgling noise as it struggles for breath. When it does slow down, it does not need as much air. The pressure is then off the whole system and the sterno-thyro-hyoideus relaxes so that the larynx can get back into its usual place and the horse can breathe again. Horses which swallow their tongues in this way are sometimes treated by surgically cutting the group of muscles which pull on the larynx. After the operation the muscles are longer by the length of scar tissue which forms, and so they do not pull as hard on the larynx.

The muscles used during breathing
Breathing is an essential bodily function, and horses, like human beings, breathe automatically. The horse breathes in by pulling each of its thirty-six ribs forwards and slightly outwards. The horse does not have to think how it is going to do this as it is controlled by an automatic nervous system. When the barrel-shaped box which the ribs make up, and which is called the thorax, is expanded in this way, the lungs are expanded as well. This is because the lungs are just the right size to fill the thorax when it is in the relaxed or breathing out position. There is a vacuum between the outer layer of the lungs and the inner wall of the thorax so that when the thorax expands it pulls the outer wall of the lungs out with it. This, in its turn, expands the body of the lung tissue. The thorax is often likened to a bellows. If you lift up the top handle of the bellows, it sucks in air. When you let it go, then it will empty the air out without any help from you. The muscles which make the horse breathe in are much more important than the muscles which make it breathe out by pulling the ribs backwards and inwards. By and large, the action of breathing out is said to be due to the natural elasticity of the lung tissue shrinking down to its 'normal' size and pulling the ribs back with it.

There are certain conditions which make it more difficult for the horse to breathe out. If this happens, the horse has to find another method to help push the air out of the lungs with more force. One way it does this is to use a muscle called the external abdominal oblique muscle. This lies across the area where the ribs end and the soft belly, or abdomen, begins. When the external abdominal oblique muscle contracts, it compresses the abdomen. This pushes the diaphragm forward and this in turn squeezes some air out of the lungs. If a horse has had to rely on its abdominal muscles to help empty its lungs, then the external abdominal oblique muscle, like all muscles which are used a great deal, increases in size. A slanting line can then be seen across the horse's abdomen where the edge of the muscle comes, and this is sometimes referred to as a 'heave line'.

The abdomen does not have a bony support such as the rib-cage provides for the abdomen. The weight of the various abdominal organs and their contents of food, liquid and faeces are supported by a muscular girdle. To be precise, the girdle is part muscle and part fibrous sheet or fascia. The largest of the muscles is the external abdominal oblique muscle. It has already been mentioned that this acts to compress the abdomen, but with its associated muscles it also supports the abdominal weight and arches the back. When just one side of the muscle contracts, it helps to bend or flex the whole body to one side. A horse which is having to use the muscle to help breathe out all the time, as may be the case if it has Chronic Obstructive Pulmonary Disease (COPD), may find difficulty in flexing its body during performance because it needs to use both sides of the muscle and not just part of it.

How the horse's back works
Most of the flexion which takes place along the horse's body is a result of the muscles of the back itself. As many kinds of poor performance have, over the years, been put down to back problems of one kind or another, it is useful to appreciate exactly what the functional anatomy of the horse's back really is. There are all sorts of fairy stories told about what can go wrong with a horse's back, and which parts of the system can move in and out of position and which cannot.

The 'back' of the horse really comprises the vertebral column itself, with its thirty-one vertebrae if the tail is not included, the large pelvis, and the muscles which join them all together. The whole can be considered to act rather like a bow kept under tension by a bowstring (Fig 3). The back is the bow and the bowstring is made up of the breast-bone, or sternum, the muscles of the abdomen and the fibrous sheets of tissue which join everything up in the midline under the body. The muscles which pull the front legs forward and those which pull the hind legs

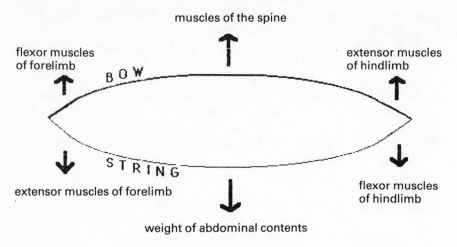

muscles of the spine

flexor muscles
of forelimb

BOW

extensor muscles
of hindlimb

STRING

extensor muscles of forelimb

flexor muscles
of hindlimb

weight of abdominal contents

Fig 3 The spinal column acting as a bow

backwards act like the muscles along the top of the back, and tend to straighten out the bow. The muscles which pull the front legs backwards and those which pull the hind legs forwards act like the abdominal muscles, and tend to keep the bow bent under tension. In the case of the horse, the bow is comparatively straight.

When a rider mounts a horse, its back does not usually sag under his weight. It is rather the opposite, in fact, because the 'bow' increases its curvature slightly. Changes in the curvature of the spine like this are achieved by contraction or relaxation of the large muscles which run along the vertebral column. The most important of these muscles, the longissimus dorsi, is the largest and longest muscle in the whole body. It runs along the top of the vertebral column all the way from the pelvis to the top of the neck.

Curvature of the back occurs gradually right along the vertebral column, and each joint between individual vertebrae hardly moves at all. The vertebrae of the lumbar region, the region behind the saddle area, are relatively inflexible. Despite the claims of chiropracters to manipulate and move individual vertebrae in this region, it is impossible to do so. Even when a horse is completely relaxed under an anaesthetic, it is impossible to move the individual vertebrae significantly, even when applying much greater force than one person could use in the conscious animal. Even after death, with the major muscles removed, it is still not possible to move individual vertebrae because of the strong ligaments which join each vertebra to the next one. The final proof of this point is that when X-rays have been taken of horses which have been claimed to have a vertebra out of alignment, they have failed to show any displacement at all.

It is when a horse jumps that we see the most movement along the vertebral column. The 'bow' is bent at take-off to provide the spring necessary for the jump. During the jump, the spring uncoils and by the time of landing the 'bow' is almost straight. When we look at a horse jumping, it appears to bend its back a great deal, but high-speed photography has shown that the vast majority of this movement actually occurs in the neck rather than along the back itself.

At this point, it might be useful to put into perspective the relative importance of the various structures of the back in so far as they cause problems to the athletic horse. One of the pioneers of research into back problems, Dr Leo Jeffcott, did a survey of nearly 450 horses with reported back problems. He found that 2.9 per cent were due to faults of conformation, 38.8 per cent were due to soft-tissue injuries affecting the muscles, ligaments, etc, and 38.6 per cent were due to problems affecting the actual bones themselves. That leaves some 19.7 per cent of the cases unaccounted for. In some of these cases it proved impossible to make a definite diagnosis, but in other cases the so-called back problem turned out to be anything from a tooth problem to a lower leg lameness!

How the horse's legs are adapted for speed of movement
The horse walks on four legs compared to our two, and this inevitably affects the way its anatomy has evolved and the varying strains which are put on the individual components. The back of the horse is obviously under a very different kind of strain from that of the human being. In our case, it is a vertical column of bones with most of the forces acting directly downwards through the column. The weight of our abdominal contents tends to pull away from our diaphragm and so does not inhibit breathing. In the case of the horse, the weight of the thoracic contents and of the abdominal contents both pull in the same direction. Extra abdominal bulk will therefore affect the movement of the diaphragm to a much greater extent than in the human being and so will make breathing more difficult. This has been recognised for centuries in the racehorse. A pail of water or a big feed just before a race can slow a horse down just as much as any chemical dope. To some extent, this makes something of a mockery of attempts to handicap horses in competitions by regulating the amount of weight which they have to carry. Some 2-3lb (0.9-1.3kg) of lead less on a horse's back will not enable it to run any faster if the horse is carrying 5lb (2.2kg) more oats in its stomach. To a large extent, the handicap system in racing has only worked because of the honesty of the trainers as generally horses are set the task of run-

ning to the best of their ability. Some trainers now place great importance on a horse's racing weight, by which they mean the weight of the
horse on its own, not its weight with a saddle, rider and weight-cloth.
They claim that results show that a horse gives its best performances at
a particular weight. This performing weight will reflect both the development of the horse's major muscle masses and the weight of its
abdominal contents.

In any consideration of the four-legged athlete compared with the
two-legged, one must remember that in the horse, not all legs are equal.
It is not just a question of 25 per cent of the horse's weight being carried
by each leg. The forelegs carry around 60 per cent of the weight when the
horse is standing or moving on level ground. This uneven distribution is
important when you are considering which leg is likeliest to be under
the greatest strain. If a leg is injured and the horse is confined to its stable for a period of time while healing takes place, there is still a lot more
strain on a front leg than there would be on a hind leg with the same
injury. Nevertheless, the healthy horse accommodates remarkably well
and if you listen to a horse trotting over a hard level surface you will
hear four completely even hoof beats. It is worth doing this from time to
time with your eyes closed because it is sometimes possible to tell when
a horse is lame with your ears before you can spot the lameness with
your eyes.

This principle has been carried a stage further (several electronic
stages further to be precise) in the Kaegi Gait Analysis System. This is a
sophisticated electronic force plate set under a hard rubber mat in an
exercise lane. The horse is walked or trotted over the unit and hundreds
of small sensors record how and when they were compressed by one of
the horse's hooves. The computer then analyses all the information and
combines it into a print-out. Even the slightest injury or strain to the
horse's locomotor system will cause a deviation from the normal pattern. The Swiss inventor of the system feels that, to some extent, it will
eliminate the need for a veterinary surgeon's diagnostic skills in detecting lameness. At the time of writing, there is comparatively little data
available on actual clinical cases and much work still remains to be
done. In any case, the cost of such equipment is high and this is likely to
restrict its availability to large research centres and a few trainers with
very rich patrons.

The horse's legs differ from those of a human being in respects other
than just having hooves. We refer to a horse's knee, but we are not talking about the same joint as a human knee. The horse's knee is the equivalent of our wrist. The cannon bone, fetlock, pastern and foot are all
developments of the third digit (our middle finger). Even the hind leg of

the horse does not correspond exactly to our leg. The stifle joint is the equivalent of our knee joint and has a knee-cap or patella like ours. The hock joint corresponds to our ankle (with the point of the hock equating to our heel), and below the hock is the third digit again.

The small splint bones which lie on either side of the cannon bone are digits which have lost their purpose and no longer bear any weight. They are not entirely functionless, however, and do help to disperse the shock waves which travel up the leg every time the horse puts its foot to the ground. If the forces of percussion are particularly strong, as when the going is very hard, or if the forces are not being directed up the centre of the cannon bone but are unevenly distributed owing to an injury, or poor conformation, then the horse may develop a splint. This is a swelling caused by the formation of new bone at some point along the ligament which binds the splint, or small metacarpal bone, to the cannon, or large metacarpal bone (Fig 4). Many horse owners expect only young horses to throw splints, but this is not necessarily the case. It is true that many young horses do throw splints, especially on the inside of

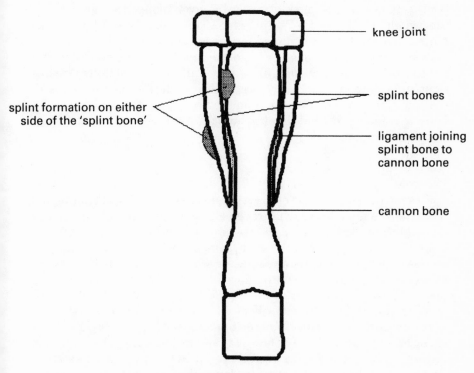

Fig 4 Splint formation

the front cannon bones, because their bone structure is too immature to withstand the forces placed upon it. The fact that the young horse is relatively unco-ordinated will also tend to mean that the concussive forces may not be as perfectly controlled as they might be. Horses of any age can throw a splint if the balance of the system is upset.

The limbs of the horse have one further peculiarity which must be mentioned before the muscle systems are dealt with in any detail. There are no muscles at all below the knee and hock joints. This is, of course, different from human beings who have fleshy muscles right down to the tips of their fingers and toes. The horse still has to control these extremities very precisely, and this means that the muscles at the top of the legs must be connected to the fetlock, pastern and foot by long tendons. The human being has no tendons of comparable length. Our Achilles tendon carries a similar workload but is only a fraction of the length of the tendons of the lower limb in the horse. The horse, incidentally, also has an Achilles tendon. It is the very thick tendon running up from the point of the hock.

The horse gallops forwards, and so the muscles of the legs have to pull the legs backwards as quickly as possible, even though they are bearing the weight of the horse at the time. This calls for well-developed muscles. When the leg is pulled forwards, on the other hand, it is not usually carrying any weight and so the muscles which do this do not have to be as well developed. They may still amount to quite sizeable structures, however. The brachiocephalic muscle, for instance, runs all the way along the horse's neck from the head to the forearm. When the horse is moving it extends the leg, but it is also the muscle which bends the neck from side to side.

Moving the front legs forward
The front leg of the horse is moved forward by two main groups of muscles. Some flex or bend the elbow and others actually pull the lower leg forward. The muscles which flex the elbow are mainly the biceps and brachialis muscles. The name biceps is, of course, familiar to all and it is interesting to note that in human beings a well-developed biceps is almost synonymous with strength for weight-lifting whereas in the horse it has only a minor role because it is only concerned with pulling the leg forward. The biceps runs from the scapula, or shoulder blade, down to the radius (the main bone in the horse's forearm above the knee). The brachialis runs from the humerus onto the radius.

The muscles which pull the lower leg forward are called the extensors, while those which pull it backwards are called the flexors. The extensor muscles of the front leg are the muscles on the front of the leg above the knee. The main muscles of this group are the extensor carpi radialis, the common digital extensor and the lateral digital extensor. They originate on the humerus or radius right at the top of the leg but they may run all the way down to the foot. The muscle fibres themselves are not that long. As has been mentioned before, there are no muscles below the knee. The rest of the distance is taken up by tendons which act rather like extension arms transferring the pulling force from the end of the muscle down to the bone which actually has to be moved. The extensor carpi radialis muscle attaches at the very top of the metacarpal, or shin, bone just below the knee. The common digital extensor muscle attaches onto the front of the phalanges, the bones which make up the pastern and foot. The lateral digital extensor muscle attaches on the front of the pastern. Backward movement of the leg starts with the pectoral muscles. These form the large fleshy mass which occupies the space between the lower chest wall and the leg. A similar function on the outer side of the leg is performed by the latissimus dorsi muscle which lies just under the skin and stretches from the withers to the forearm.

Moving the front legs backwards
The horse's elbow is extended, or straightened, mainly by the triceps muscle. This is a large muscle which, as its name implies, divides into three parts. So, part of the triceps comes from the scapula and two parts come from the humerus. They all join together and attach at the same place, the olecranon. This is the point of the elbow.

The lower part of the front leg is pulled backwards by the flexor muscles. These comprise the medial flexor of the carpus, the lateral flexor of the carpus, the superficial digital flexor and the deep digital flexor. Of these, the superficial and deep flexors are the most important because these are the muscles which move the foot and therefore need to have long tendons to transfer their pull down to the very end of the leg. When people talk about a horse's tendons they often just mean the superficial and deep tendons. They can be felt very easily where they run down the back of the metacarpus, or cannon bone, below the knee. They make up the first cord of tendon which you can feel. If you feel carefully, you can find the division into the superficial and deep portions. The other cord of tendon tissue which you can feel between the flexor tendons and the metacarpal bone is not really tendon at all. It is the suspensory ligament. The difference between tendons and ligaments is really quite simple. Tendons, as has been explained, are really extensions of muscles and are therefore involved in moving things. Ligaments join two bones together, to hold them in place, and are not involved in actually moving the bones. The front leg of the horse has, then, a dual system of opposing muscles which enables it to place its foot on the ground and pull it backwards while it is bearing the horse's weight. The leg is then raised and moved forwards ready for the next cycle. It is obvious that the foot does not actually move backwards over the surface of the ground; rather, it stays stationary while the horse's body is propelled forwards until it looks as if the leg has been moved backwards.

The stay apparatus

If that was all there was to the system there would be a very weak position when the horse was standing. The extensors and flexors would balance each other out, but there would be nothing actually holding the horse up. The horse has therefore developed a mechanism called the stay apparatus which enables it to stand firmly without excessive ten-

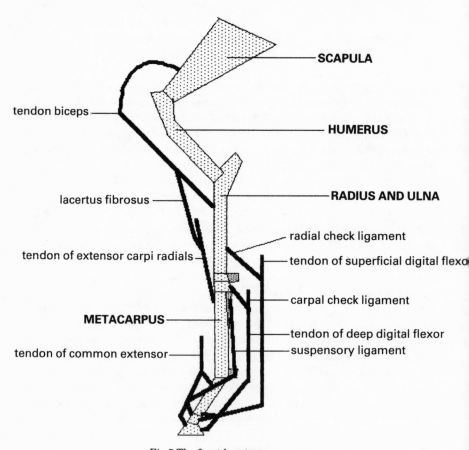

Fig 5 The front leg stay apparatus

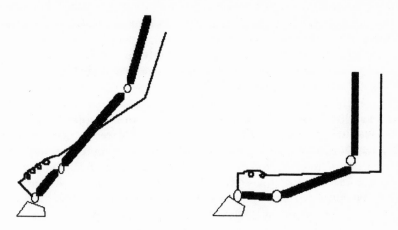

Fig 6 The spring action of the suspensory ligament

sion in the muscles of the leg, and even enables it to go to sleep standing up (Fig 5). The tendon of the superficial digital flexor is given a 'check ligament' which links the tendon to the radius bone. The check ligament prevents the tendon from being pulled too far down when the fetlock is bearing weight, and so helps to prevent the fetlock collapsing down onto the ground. The deep flexor tendon is also provided with a check ligament. This is called the carpal check ligament and it links the deep flexor tendon to the carpal, or knee, bones. If the flexor tendons are completely ruptured during really strenuous exercise, then the fetlock does indeed collapse completely (Plate 3).

The suspensory ligament is the other part of the stay apparatus. It starts at the knee, attached to the back of the knee and the top part of the cannon bone. As has been mentioned, it then runs down the back of the cannon bone, between the bone and the flexor tendons. Just above the fetlock joint, it divides into two. Each branch of the suspensory ligament attaches onto one of the two sesamoid bones at the fetlock joint and then continues forward to join the extensor tendon on the front of the pastern. It therefore provides a link between the flexor and extensor systems, literally suspending the fetlock joint. Fig 6 shows how the branches of the suspensory ligament act like another 'bowstring' for the fetlock joint. When the horse's weight takes the fetlock joint down, the 'bow' is bent, ready to snap straight and give some impulsion to the leg. The suspensory ligament continues down past the fetlock in the form of the distal sesamoidean ligaments. These link the sesamoid bones with the first and second phalanges, the bones of the pastern.

The anatomy of the foot and lower leg

The conformation of the fetlock and pastern can readily affect the chances of a horse suffering from conditions such as ringbone and sesamoiditis. The sesamoid bones, incidentally, are two in number and lie right at the back of the fetlock joint. They are shaped rather like pyramids. They are extra bones which are not part of the main column of the leg which has to withstand the stresses and strains of bearing the horse's weight. Instead, they act rather as a fulcrum, enabling the flexor tendons and the suspensory ligament to change direction from vertically downwards to forwards. Sesamoiditis is an inflammation of the sesamoid bones owing to too much pull being exerted on the ligaments and tendons which attach onto them. Where the ligaments, etc, pull on the surface of the periosteum, or surface of the bone, new bone is often formed. As is often the case when this happens, it can be painful and cause lameness. In some cases the ligaments may even pull a chip of bone off the sesamoid bone, and such a fracture will certainly cause problems.

If a horse has upright pasterns, it increases the compression of the column of bones up the leg. In other words, all the percussion forces which have to be absorbed by the leg when the foot hits the ground have to be coped with by the bones themselves; the stay apparatus and the tendons cannot provide much 'give' or springing. The opposite is the case with a horse which has very sloping pasterns. The flexor tendons and the suspensory ligament are then stretched more than normal, and fast work etc may easily result in sprained tendons or sesamoiditis.

There is another sesamoid bone in the lower leg, the distal sesamoid bone. Although that name may not be familiar, most horse owners have heard of it under its more common name of the navicular bone. It lies behind the pedal bone, or third phalanx, and the second phalanx (Fig 7). Looked at from the side, it looks rather like a wedge, and it fits neatly between the other two bones. Just as the sesamoid bones of the fetlock joint act as a fulcrum for changing the direction of tendons, so does the navicular bone. The deep flexor tendon runs over the rear surface of the navicular bone before it attaches onto the back of the pedal bone.

For such a small bone, hidden away in the horse's foot, the navicular bone causes a great deal of trouble. Navicular disease is probably the most important cause of chronic lameness in the horse. It appears that the condition arises because of venous congestion in the blood-vessels of the foot. Because the blood cannot pass through the foot as quickly as it should, the actual blood pressure in the foot goes up. The pain associated with navicular disease is thought to be due to this rise in pressure in the blood-vessels. This explains why, for example, bending the foot hard back at the fetlock joint makes horses with navicular disease so lame. The procedure has been shown to further increase the pressure in the blood-vessels of the foot. Some of the congested vessels in the actual bone itself may develop an arteriosclerosis. The associated blood clot blocks the vessel, preventing it from being of any further use. Unless the horse can quickly start to make another blood-vessel and push this into the navicular bone to supply that area of the bone, it will start to die. Dying bone is painful bone, and this adds to the lameness.

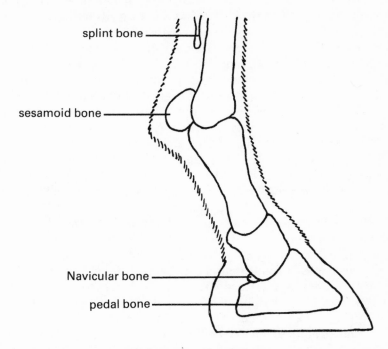

Fig 7 The bones of the lower leg

So far, we do not know why some horses are more susceptible to navicular disease, ie why some horses have a poorer blood flow through their feet than others. We do know some of the contributing factors, though. Breed appears to have some effect, with Thoroughbred crosses especially likely to have the disease and ponies far less likely. Conformation also has an effect. This may be natural conformation, with long sloping pasterns causing greater than normal strain in the deep flexor tendon. More commonly, artificially altered conformation is involved. Poor shoeing can alter the angle of the foot and so likewise increase the pressure which the tendon exerts, pressing the navicular bone into the space between the other two bones. If the horse's toe is allowed to grow too long while the heels are cut too short, then the horse is much more likely to develop navicular disease.

Navicular disease usually affects both front feet to a greater or lesser extent, but the horse may only appear lame on one front leg (presumably the leg which hurts it the most). It is relatively rare for the condition to affect the hind feet. It is possible for a horse not to appear lame with navicular disease but just to have a shortening of its stride or a decrease in its performance. When the horse's feet are X-rayed (perhaps when the horse is examined prior to sale) the characteristic signs can, however, be seen (Plate 4). We do not know why some horses can stand quite marked changes in their navicular bone without showing any clinical signs of lameness, whereas other horses will go lame with navicular disease even before the bony changes are sufficiently advanced to show on an X-ray plate. It may, however, be related to variations in the pain thresholds of the different horses to the increased blood pressure.

Treatment of navicular disease has now advanced past the stage of merely reducing the pain or killing the animal. It is possible to use drugs which specifically improve the blood supply to the bone. Warfarin will do this by increasing the flexibility of the red blood cells so that they can pass more readily through the narrow blood-vessels. It does, however, also increase the time taken for blood to clot throughout the whole body. Great care, therefore, must be taken to check the horse's blood-clotting time throughout the period of treatment in order to ensure that its life is not in danger from a small wound causing a fatal haemorrhage. Isoxsuprine will increase the blood supply to the whole foot because it is what is known as a peripheral vasodilator. It does not increase the blood-clotting time, and so does not need such careful monitoring. At the present time, results in the UK would indicate that about 80 per cent of horses treated with warfarin will return to work, and about 50 per cent of horses treated with isoxsuprine will do so. Work is continuing all over the world to evaluate the different methods of treatment, however, and not everyone would agree with these figures.

The muscles of the horse's hind quarters are often looked upon as the power-house for its performance. Again, the muscles to the front of the leg, which pull it forward through the air, are less important and less well developed than the muscles at the back of the leg. There are four main joints along the hind leg: the hip joint, the stifle, the hock and the fetlock. They are all cross-linked together so that it is difficult to move one of them without moving all the others. The leg is rather like an extending ladder with alternate joints bending in opposite directions when the leg is raised. This is different from human beings who can move their foot, for example, without moving their knee or hip joints.

When we look at a horse in competitive conditions, it is possible to pick out the superficial muscles of its hind leg underneath its skin. Stretching down from the tuber coxae (which is the bony prominence just behind the flanks and which is part of the pelvis and not, as so many people seem to think, the horse's hip) is the tensor fascia latae muscle which attaches around the stifle. Immediately above this is the superficial gluteal muscle. They both flex the hip joint. The hip joint itself can be felt on the horse, but it is covered with muscle and is not immediately obvious. There are actually three gluteal muscles. They form one of the most important muscle masses in the horse, not least because of their role in propelling the horse forwards by moving the hind leg. Behind the tensor fascia latae and superficial gluteal muscles is a curved muscle which appears to run from the spine down to the stifle joint. This is the biceps femoris (which should not be confused with the biceps brachii of the front leg). Despite its name, it has three bellies of muscle, not two. The muscle right at the back of the hind leg is the semitendinosus. These two muscles extend the leg, which means that they move the horse's body forward when the foot is fixed by being on the ground. They also push the leg out behind the horse, thus enabling it to rear, jump or kick. They are, therefore, important muscles to the owner of an athletic horse in more ways than one.

The large muscle masses at the back of the thigh, comprising the biceps femoris, semitendinosus, semimembranosus and gracilis muscles have another significance apart from their role in movement. If a horse develops azoturia (which is also known as set-fast or tying-up syndrome), then it often involves these muscles and they become hard and painful to the touch. This is not because of their anatomical position but because of their sheer size, as will be discussed later.

At first glance, the leg below the horse's stifle appears to be an exception to the rule that the muscles at the back of the leg, pulling it backwards, are better developed than those in front of the leg. The two muscles which can be 'seen' are at the front and are the long digital extensor and the lateral digital extensor. These muscles, plus the tibialis anterior muscle, extend the leg forwards. The muscles which flex the leg are actually no less well developed, but are higher up the leg, almost under the muscle of the thigh. As in the front leg, there are superficial and deep digital flexor muscles and their tendons. There is also the gastrocnemius muscle. This is a powerful muscle which ends in the gastrocnemius tendon, otherwise known as the Achilles or calcaneal tendon. The gastrocnemius tendon fastens onto the tuber calcis, the bone which forms the point of the hock. The superficial flexor tendon also passes over the point of the tuber calcis, on top of the gastrocnemius tendon, and it is this tendon (and not the gastrocnemius) which can sometimes 'slip off' the hock during violent exercise.

The hind leg also needs a stay apparatus to enable the back half of the horse to have some rigidity. Below the hock the anatomy is, to all intents and purposes, exactly the same as the front leg, but above the hock there are some significant differences. The tensor fascia latae muscle has already been mentioned as attaching onto the patella, or knee cap, as a sheet of fibrous tissue, or fascia. The patella forms a vital part of the stay apparatus.

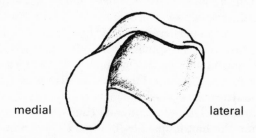

medial   lateral

Fig 8 The medial edge of the diamond-shaped patella forms a 'hook' which can be locked over the femur in order to fix the whole hind leg rigid. Note how smooth this posterior surface of the bone is so that it moves smoothly over the femur and tibia during movement.

The patella itself is basically diamond shaped, but when seen from the rear (the part which moves over the femur), it has a definite hook (Fig 8). Three strong ligaments run down from the patella. One starts from this hook of cartilage, which is on the medial side of the bone when it is in place on the horse's leg, one from the bottom of the diamond and one from the outside, or lateral, corner. When the horse is standing still it locks the hook of cartilage over a bony 'peg' on the bottom of the femur, and this keeps the patella fixed at its uppermost limit of movement. Because the three ligaments from the patella all fasten onto a ridge on the front of the tibia, this effectively locks the whole leg. If one joint of the leg is locked, then the other joints will not readily move either. When the horse wants to move off, it gets the tensor fascia latae muscle to contract and slightly lift the patella. The hook of the patella is then freed, and the patella is able to move freely up and down over a groove in the end of the femur.

Occasionally, something goes wrong with the system. The patella locks in position, but the horse is unable to free it and so is unable to bend the leg. The horse may then be seen moving around dragging the rigid leg behind it. This happens when the medial patellar ligament is a fraction too short so that the tensor fascia latae is not quite able to pull the patella off the femoral ridge. If a horse or pony is allowed to lose a lot of condition, then a general loss of elasticity in its ligaments and tendons can result in this upward fixation, or locking, of the patella. It can also arise as a result of injury. The commonest way for this to happen is for the horse to over-extend its hind leg behind itself, common during jumping or kicking, and so strain the ligament. The resulting inflammation shortens the ligament.

Treatment of the inflammation in such cases with anti-inflammatory drugs will often lead to a speedy cure for the condition. Where this fails, surgery is necessary. The medial ligament is cut completely but then allowed to heal. When it does so, it is effectively lengthened by the width of the scar tissue which forms, and this lengthening is sufficient to allow the patella to move freely once again. If a horse does suffer a locked patella during a competition, incidentally, do not attempt to bend the leg. The stifle should be massaged and an attempt made to manouevre the patella 'off the hook' before bending the leg, otherwise you will pull the ligaments even further.

The rest of the stay apparatus in the hind leg is basically the same as that of the front leg. The deep digital flexor tendon of the hind leg has a check ligament (the tarsal check ligament because the term tarsal is used for everything to do with the hock in the same way as carpal is used for the knee) just as that of the front leg has. The superficial digital flexor does not, however, have a check ligament equivalent to the radial check ligament.

No account of the horse's anatomy, however brief, would be complete without looking at the hoof. The horse's hoof consists of a semicircular wall, which is roughly equivalent to our nail, and a flat sole. It is made from horn, a versatile substance which can vary in hardness from the hard hoof wall to the soft horn of the frog. Looked at under a microscope, horn appears as thousands of tubules bound together in a 'cement'. The tubules grow downwards from either the coronet or the inner surface of the sole. They vary slightly in structure from the inside of the hoof out to the surface. Horse owners over the years have speculated why some hooves crack easier than others or seem generally weaker than others, and it has been suggested that this might be due to differences in the pigment granules which give the horn its colour. This is not the case. Light-coloured horn is no weaker than dark horn. If it was then horses with bands of light and dark horn in a hoof would find the two 'types' of horn shearing away from each other. There is no point, therefore, in selecting a horse for good feet which will stand up to the strain of competition partly on the basis of the amount of pigment in the horn. The major factor which affects horn strength is its moisture content. This is partly genetic and partly affected by stable management. Keeping a horse standing in damp bedding will not help it to have strong horn, especially if the outer waterproofing layer has been rasped away during shoeing.

New horn is continually being formed by the stratum germinativum cells in the coronary band and under the sole of the hoof, and this lengthens the horn tubules. The tubules themselves are not a living tissue which can repair itself. If the tubules are distorted in shape by poor foot trimming, they cannot right themselves. Even after the fault has been corrected, you will have to wait for new horn to grow down before you will see any improvement. Similarly, cracks will not seal themselves; all you can do is to prevent any movement of the crack edges which might perpetuate the condition, and wait for the crack to grow out.

Where the hoof and the rest of the foot are attached, there are thousands of minute finger-like projections from one into the other. These are, in turn, arranged on microscopic folds which are called the sensitive laminae. The hoof is therefore held onto the foot in rather a similar way to the interlocking of a jigsaw puzzle. There is a plexus, or network, of tiny blood-vessels between the hoof and the bone. Any inflammation or alteration of the blood supply which causes dilation of these capillaries will make the horse's foot very painful because the horn is too rigid to allow the blood-vessels to swell. This is the situation in laminitis. Although laminitis is only part of a condition which affects the whole body, it is the set of symptoms which is most likely to come to the owner's attention. What happens is that carbohydrates taken into the horse's stomach cause a variety of changes elsewhere in the body, including the release of histamine-type chemicals. Perhaps the major result of this is a stasis, or slowing of the blood flow, in the circulation away from the feet. Not only do the feet then become warm and painful, but the reduced blood flow also interferes, in the long term, with the production of healthy horn. Although exercise is important in the treatment of a horse with laminitis, the very first step should be to empty out the existing contents of the alimentary tract in order to remove the root cause of the problem. Poor shoeing, and other factors which adversely affect the blood flow through the horse's feet, will also increase the likelihood or severity of an attack of laminitis.

From the point of view of the athletic horse, the end result of the physical anatomy in the foot is that the total weight of the horse (which may be 880lb (400kg) in a Thoroughbred but up to 1,320lb (600kg) in an eventer) is supported internally by a large surface area of sensitive laminae which is packed into the relatively small volume of the foot.

This same system, where the hoof is in interlocking contact with the sensitive parts of the foot but is not part of them, allows the horn to grow while the pedal bone, etc, remain in the same position. If this were not so, the horn could not slide very slowly over the outer surface of the sensitive laminae as the hoof grows down from the coronary band, only to be worn away by friction during exercise.

How joints work

Muscles, tendons and ligaments would be useless without a system of moving joints. Practically all of these have the same basic structure, although their shape and anatomy may vary. The surfaces of the bones which are going to be in contact with each other are covered with a smooth cartilage; it is never actually bone moving on bone. The joint has a sleeve around it composed of the fibrous joint capsule and a lining of synovial membrane. The joint cavity is filled with synovial fluid, or joint fluid. This is a thick, clear amber liquid. It is thixotropic, which means that when it is being disturbed by the movements of the bones in the joint, it becomes quite thin in order to provide as little resistance to movement as possible. Away from the moving bone surfaces, however, it is relatively thick. In other words, it is rather like non-drip paint in its behaviour. The lubricant properties of synovial fluid come largely from a substance called hyaluronic acid. Not only is this present in the fluid, it is also incorporated into the cartilage as well. It really is an efficient low-friction system within the joints.

Hard training may result in excessive wear on the cartilage of any of a horse's joints. This wear releases chemicals into the joint which reduce the levels of hyaluronic acid in the synovial fluid. At the same time, the synovial membrane is making increased amounts of synovial fluid. The wise trainer promptly reduces the workload of such a horse, which allows things to return to normal. If the joint is subjected to further stresses, the damage will progress until the cartilage is eroded right through so that bare bone is exposed. This is very painful and requires prolonged rest to allow healing. Not all erosions of the cartilage are necessarily associated with lameness. Using an instrument called an arthroscope, we can insert a flexible viewing tube into a joint and see the results of wear and tear in the living, active horse. If, however, we look at the joints of perfectly sound horses after death we will still see these erosions even though the horse was never lame.

Replacing the increased amount of substandard synovial fluid with either good quality fluid from a healthy joint on the same horse, or with artificially synthesised hyaluronic acid, will quickly restore normal function to many of these 'filled' joints. The horse can then return to work almost immediately. In the search for a drug which will enable a rapid return to work in such situations, corticosteroids have, in the past, often been injected directly into the joints. Their anti-inflammatory action has, as will be seen in a later chapter, been very effective. Unfortunately, there have often been disastrous side effects at a later date because corticosteroids can have major effects on bone. It would not be exaggerating too much to say that when an intra-articular injection of corticosteroid has gone wrong, the joint has almost literally collapsed.

There is now a tendency to call such conditions an 'arthrosis' rather than arthritis. To some extent this reflects that it is the joint itself which is degenerating rather than being a problem which is triggered off by new bone growth. This realisation that it is cartilage breakdown which occurs first has come hand in hand with the development of arthroscopy in the horse. This is a technique where a narrow flexible tube is inserted into the joint. The surgeon can then look along thousands of glass fibres which lie in the tube and see exactly what is going on inside the joint. The tip of the arthroscope can be moved in any direction in order to explore the whole joint. Previously, our knowledge had been based on post mortem examinations, which inevitably were old established cases (often where the disease had progressed so much that the horse was permanently lame and so was euthanased). It seemed logical to imagine that new bone would irritate the joint, and it was impossible to detect which disease process had come first. Arthroscopy has changed that, and enabled us to see what is going on in even early cases. It has also given us the means of removing pieces of floating bone (called bone mice), etc from joints without resorting to major open-joint surgery.

It is obvious from all that has gone before in this chapter that the structure of the horse is a mixture of general principles and specific adaptations. The foot of the horse is the same basic structure whether it is a front foot or a hind foot. It is even the same whether it is a left front foot or a right front foot. There are marked similarities between the stay apparatus of the front legs and that of the hind legs, but there are also marked differences. It is possible, for instance, to pick up a front foot and bend it backwards at the knee without moving the leg above the knee. It is not, on the other hand, possible to pick up a hind foot without moving the leg above the hock. When one looks at the major muscles of movement, however, the muscle masses have a completely different anatomy in the front and hind legs. The body as a whole is organised into an efficient machine which can move exceedingly quickly when racing, but also very precisely in dressage. It is rare for a horse to excel at more than one of the many varied disciplines simply because it is rare to find a horse which is physically and mentally built to do so. Just as there is often a lack of versatility in the human athlete, with few gymnasts, for example, also excelling as marathon runners, so it is with horses. It depends on a mixture of conformation and genetic attributes whether training, however skilled and prolonged, will develop your horse's suppleness, power or endurance in the field at which you want it to excel.

2 · How the Horse Moves

When we walk we take it for granted that our legs will move one after the other. When we run we take it for granted that they will move in the same order but much faster. The horse is much more complicated. It moves its four legs in different orders depending on which speed or type of movement is required. Each order of leg movement is called a gait. It has been shown that there is a natural transition from one gait to another in order to use the horse's energy most efficiently. Although there are four 'natural' gaits (the walk, trot, canter and gallop), there are also artificial gaits, such as the pace. These have been developed in particular strains or breeds of horse which first showed a tendency to break into such a gait for a few strides. The result is that, after decades of breeding and selection, the artificial gait is almost second nature to that particular breed and it will hopefully take very little training to develop it to the point where the trained horse will break into, say, the pace when commanded to do so. There are even some breeds where a particular gait, the pace, for example, is no longer considered to be artificial but is part of the genetic make-up of the breed. The walk, trot, canter and gallop remain, however, the gaits which all horses, whether Standardbred or Thoroughbred, Shetland Pony or Draught Horse, can and do perform.

When a leg is moved during locomotion, it can be said to have two phases, or functional activities. It is either in the stance phase, during which it is in contact with the ground and bearing weight to some degree, or in the swing phase, during which it is lifted off the ground and moved forward ready to be placed on the ground again. Until the camera was sufficiently developed to 'freeze' the movement of a horse's legs on a photographic plate, people were handicapped in any attempt to find out which leg moved where and when by the difficulty of telling when the leg was picked up from the ground, ie when it entered the swing phase. As early as 1779, two Frenchmen, Goiffon and Vincent, tied bells onto each of a horse's legs and tried to determine the order of movement during the trot, pace and gallop. Using such crude methods, it was possible to tell that successive strides used the legs in the same order and that in some gaits, eg the walk, trot and pace, the legs on the left and right sides

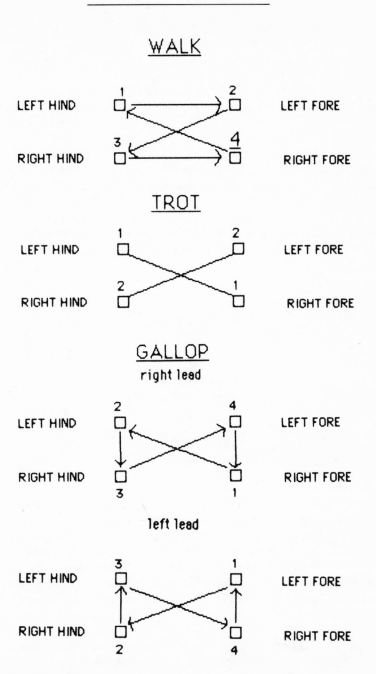

Fig 9 The gaits of the horse. The numbers and arrows show the order in which the horse puts its feet to the ground

of the horse moved symmetrically but that in others, eg the canter and gallop, they did not.

The original photographs of the horse in motion were taken using twelve or twenty-four still cameras triggered off in sequence. In 1877 Professor Muybridge in America filmed a trotter at the racing trot and showed for the very first time there were moments when the horse was completely suspended in the air, without any feet touching the ground. Since that time the still camera has been superseded by first the ordinary movie camera and more recently by ultra-high-speed cinematography taking five hundred or more frames per second. It has not been abandoned completely, however, because the 'photo-finish', where a single picture taken at the exact moment when the first part of a horse passes the winning post in a race determines which horse has won, is still in use all over the world from the Epsom Derby down to the lowliest selling, or claiming, race.

The walk

The slowest gait is the walk. The horse picks up its left hind foot and moves it forward. As it does so it picks up the left front foot, so that at this stage there are only two feet on the ground (both on the right side of the animal). The left hind foot is then placed on the ground, followed by the left front foot. As the left front foot is being placed down, however, the right hind leg is being lifted up. The right front foot is raised as the right hind foot is being brought forward (so that there are only two feet on the ground again). The right hind foot is then put to the ground, followed by the right front foot (Fig 9).

The trot

In the trot the horse is alternately balanced on diagonally opposite feet. The horse picks up both the right hind and the left front feet. As it places these to the ground again it picks up the left hind and right front feet (Fig 9). It is because the trot is such a balanced and symmetrical gait that it is so invaluable in showing whether a horse is lame or not. At any one time the horse has one front leg and one hind leg bearing weight. In a front leg lameness the horse's head will nod downwards when it bears

Plate 1 The Successful Event Horse – *Priceless*, ridden by Virginia Holgate, at the water jump whilst winning the 1985 European Three Day Event (Courtesy Stuart Newsham)

Plate 2 (*overleaf*) The Successful Racehorse – *Sharastani*, ridden by Walter Swinburn, winning the 1986 Epsom Derby (Courtesy Sports & General Press Agency)

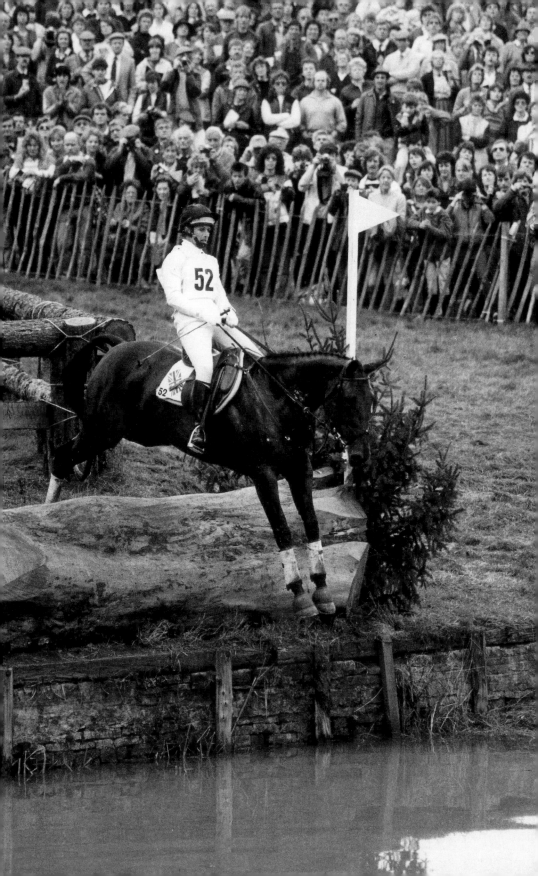

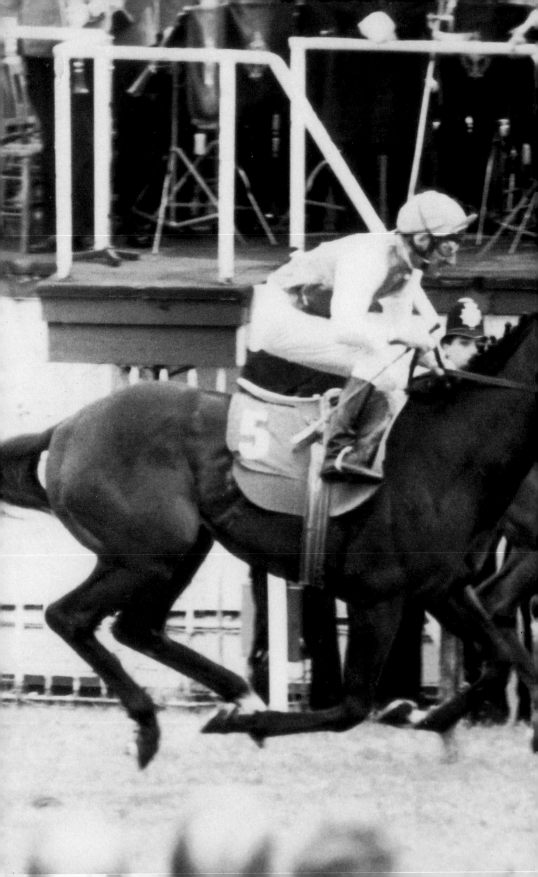

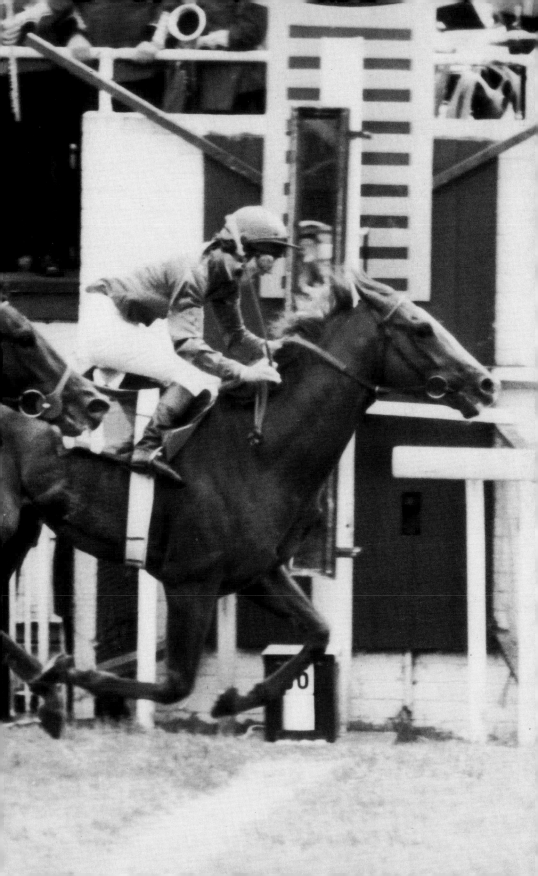

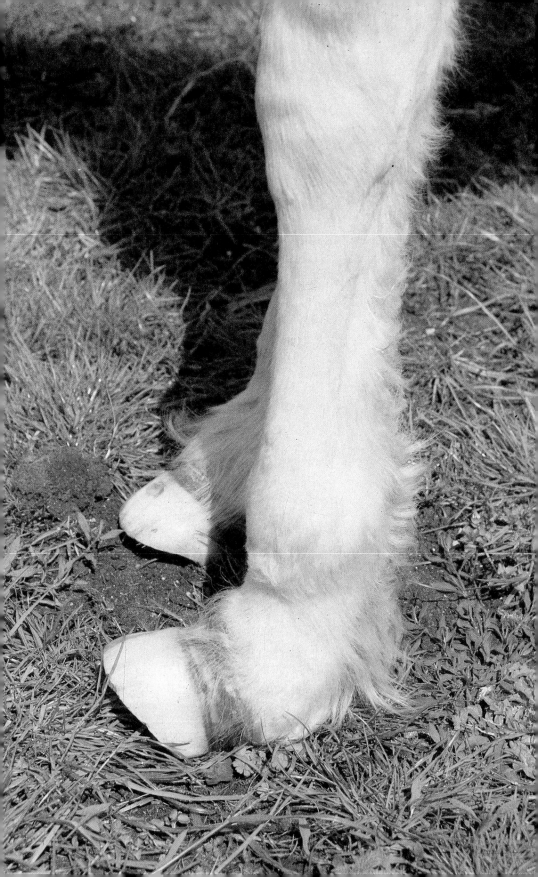

extra weight on the good front leg, and so it is lame on the opposite front leg. In a hind leg lameness the horse's rump will sink when it bears extra weight on the good hind leg. Occasionally, the inexperienced eye may be slightly confused and think that a horse is lame on the diametrically opposite leg to the one that is actually causing the trouble, ie the leg which is bearing weight at the same time as the one which is showing pain.

The canter

The canter and gallop are very similar gaits. Both have two possible leg sequences, according to which leg is the leading leg. When a horse leads with its right front leg, it is that leg which throws the horse into the floating phase which Professor Muybridge showed in his early photographs. The horse then lands on its left hind leg, and the right hind leg follows. In the canter, these two legs remain on the ground while the left front leg also comes to bear weight. The left and then the right hind legs are then lifted up, leaving only the left front foot on the ground. At this stage the horse throws its right front leg forwards and this takes over from the left front leg as the only weight-bearing leg, ready to throw the horse into the suspension phase again (Fig 9). When the horse leads with its left front leg, it then lands on first the right hind leg and then the left hind leg. These are followed by the right front leg before the left front leg throws the horse into the suspension phase again (Fig 9). When a horse is galloping, the increased speed means that both the hind legs are basically off the ground by the time that the first front leg is coming to bear weight. The result is that whereas in the canter there is a time when there are three legs on the ground at the same time, at the gallop there are only ever two legs on the ground at any one time. In fact, it is a general principle that the faster the horse is travelling, the fewer the number of legs there are supporting it. If we consider the trot to be a gait in two time, the canter is in three time, whereas the gallop appears to the rider to be in four time.

When the horse is moving at speed, it is the heel and angle of the hoof wall which are the first part of the foot to come in contact with the ground. This is the situation in thoroughbreds and standardbreds at any rate. At slow speeds, however, the foot is placed down flatly, with the whole of the bearing surface hitting the ground at the same time. This means that when a horse is travelling at speed, at the point of impact the flexor tendons are already under tension, and the impact itself will place even greater strain on them. It might also mean that calkins

Plate 3 A horse with ruptured flexor tendons

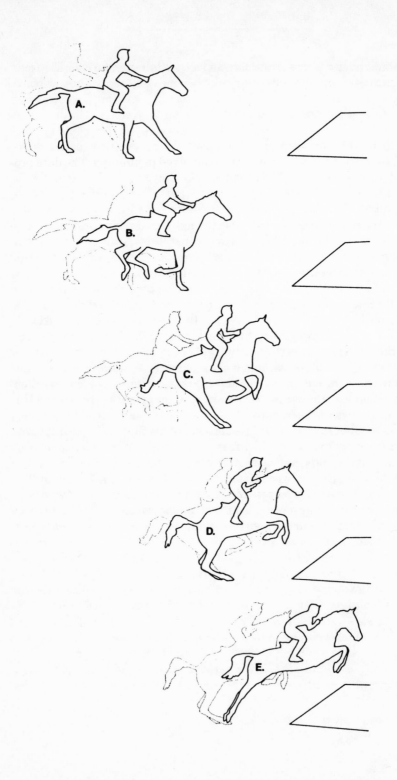

and studs placed at the heels of the shoes reduce even further the cross-sectional area which takes this first strain, giving a relatively unstable situation.

Jumping

Recent studies in Canada using high speed cinematography have led to increased information on the actions involved in jumping. The data produced dispels some popularly held beliefs. Contrary to the normal view, it has been found that the forelimbs have a very important role in generating the initial vertical forces necessary. The strutting action of the forelimbs changes the momentum of forward movement into vertical impulse. The hindlimbs have a synchronous and symmetrical action at takeoff which allows the limbs to co-ordinate their movement in the air phase (Fig 10).

The forces of movement

When the foot first hits the ground, it has a braking effect on the movement of that particular leg, and indeed of the whole horse. This decelerating force acts horizontally, parallel to the ground. It lasts relatively longer for hind legs than it does for front legs. As the leg becomes vertical, it bears more of the horse's weight until the maximum vertical force is being borne by the leg when it is completely vertical. At this stage the leg movement has only succeeded in slowing the horse down and in keeping it supported; it still has not made it go any faster. The function of the final part of the stance phase is to exert an accelerating force, again parallel to the ground and in the direction of travel. If a horse is travelling at a steady speed, the decelerating forces have to equal the accelerating forces. When we are considering the horse as an athlete, we naturally tend to think of the accelerating force as the most important. In fact, the leg does not spend the majority of its time in contact with the ground on this accelerating force. It is the decelerating

---

Fig 10 Traced outline showing selected stages of take-off during a steeplechase jump. A) initial placement of lead left foreleg on the ground. Both hindlimbs are still in the swing phase. B) the recoil from the forelimbs begins to elevate the forequarters and the hindlimbs are drawn under the body. C) initial synchronous contact of the hindlimbs on the ground. At this phase, the forequarters are still moving vertically and the hindlimbs are not capable of horizontal propulsion. D) phase when the hindlimbs start to generate horizontal and vertical propulsion, since the hip joint has moved past the ground contact point of the hoof. Prior to this (between C and D), the horse would be generating decelerating forces, E) final propulsive effort of the hindlimbs. The body does not elevate appreciably after this phase (from the technique of jumping a steeplechase fence by competing event horses, D. H. Leach and K. Omerod. Appl. Animal Behaviour Sciences *12* 15-24 (1984))

force which occupies more of the time, 40-45 per cent of the stance phase. It is also interesting that the amount of weight which the leg (and so the flexor tendons) has to bear varies with the speed and gait which the horse is using. At the walk the peak vertical force is 0.6 of the body-weight. This increases to 0.9-1.0 of the body-weight at the trot. By the time the horse reaches the gallop, each leg is having to withstand a force equal to 1.75 of the horse's body-weight every time it reaches the point of peak vertical force. We are starting to see why it is hardly surprising that tendons fail to stand up to all this and become injured. There is evidence that some horses may subconsciously prefer to use one leg more than another. When they do this the horizontal forces, both of acceleration and deceleration will no longer be equal for all four legs. This might well affect such a horse's performance, and might even in the long run contribute to the development of lameness.

A horse's stride length is measured as the distance between consecutive footfalls of the same leg. A variety of factors can influence stride length. Variations in the horse's height and the length of its limbs will obviously affect it. It is also known that the weight of the horse-shoes and the weight of any cart, eg a sulky which the horse is pulling, can also affect the stride length. The weight of the rider, on the other hand, does not appear to alter it. This is not as contradictory as it might at first seem. The weight of the shoes and the weight of a cart will affect the horizontal forces on the leg, whereas the weight of a rider will affect the vertical forces. The individual horse maintains a more or less constant stride length at any one speed, even when this is measured on several different occasions. Individual horses within a breed, even horses of almost identical size and conformation, may, however, show marked variation in stride length at identical speeds. A racing trotter's stride length will be about 6yd (5.45m) long. A horse at the pace may have a stride length of 7½yd (7m), almost as long as the 7½-8½yd (7-8m) stride length of a galloping horse. Despite these variations in stride length, the stride duration, which is the time taken for a single stride, remains approximately the same (just under half a second).

The velocity of any moving object is, as any schoolboy knows, its rate of motion. In the case of an athlete it is equivalent to the stride length multiplied by the stride frequency. The stride length of a human sprinter does not increase as fast as his stride frequency when he is approaching his maximum speed. In other words, if he is to go any faster he needs to obtain a relatively greater increase in his stride frequency. It used to be thought that when a horse was galloping, its stride frequency was more or less constant even if it was galloping faster and faster. This would have meant that the horse, unlike the human athlete, obtained its increased speed by increasing its stride length. We now know that both frequency and length of stride are important in the horse. When a horse is moving at speeds of up to 547yd (500m) per minute, increased speed comes from an increase in stride length. At speeds of over 766yd (700m) per minute, such acceleration comes from increase in stride frequency. So, the galloping horse increases its speed by taking more strides per minute, and decreases its speed by taking less. Once it has reached the desired speed, it maintains it by increasing (or decreasing) its stride length, and this then allows it to alter its stride frequency back towards its original rate. We expect a horse to be able to gallop faster when it has been subjected to a training programme, and it is interesting that training has been shown to increase stride length. Presumably, this is part of the reason why it increases the horse's maximum speed.

There are a variety of subtle changes which occur in a horse's gait as it becomes tired or fatigued. The racing Thoroughbred, for example, starts to allow the stance phase of its legs to overlap, especially those of the leading hind leg and the non-leading front leg. Such overlaps may well predispose the horse to injuries at the end of a race. The tired horse may also alter the timing of its stride in order to decrease the total weight-bearing responsibility of its lead hind leg and non-lead front leg. If, in the future, it were to become possible to measure readily such changes out on the practice gallops, we would be in a position to assess the success of various training methods in delaying the onset of fatigue.

The different gaits each have a different metabolic requirement from the body – they require differing amounts of oxygen and energy to propel the horse along at the same velocity. Left to its own inclinations, the horse appears to change its gait at the speed which will be most economical in the demands which it places on the body. It is rather like the mini-computers which are now built into some modern cars to tell the driver his precise petrol consumption, etc at any one time, so that he can drive as economically as possible. Even within a certain gait the horse may ring the changes. If it changes its leading front leg while galloping, the horse will reduce fatigue. It does this by changing its leg order immediately after the suspension phase. There is nothing wrong with lead changes as such, but if they are performed inefficiently they may reduce the overall speed.

Not surprisingly, the surface on which the horse is asked to work will affect its strides. A sandy surface will force a horse to reduce both its stride length and its frequency compared with when it is performing over solid ground. Going which allows the horse's foot to penetrate the surface introduces another dimension to our forces. The peak vertical force will remain the same, but the horizontal forces will also increase in magnitude. The total vertical force reflects how deep the foot is sinking into the surface and how readily it does so. The result is that on soft going either the velocity of the horse is reduced or it has to use much more force and energy to compensate and so maintain the original velocity. As the horse gets tired it may not be able to compensate, and will run slower and slower. Working a horse up and down hills is rather similar. The horizontal forces are altered by the fact that the foot is at a different height when it is replaced on the ground than it was when it was lifted up. Extra effort is naturally required to enable the horse to cover a set distance up or down a hill compared with moving over flat ground. It is the physical forces acting on the individual feet that cause this, not just the fact of lifting the horse another couple of inches above sea-level. If it was just lifting that required extra effort, then going down-hill would require very little effort at all, and this is just not the case.

Initially, the sole effect of fatigue is to make the horse run slower or perform less accurately. If the horse continues to ask its muscles for more effort, then problems arise which will be discussed elsewhere. The co-ordination of the system of movement also begins to deteriorate, and this results in excessive strains being placed on some components of the system. Eventually, one of these components may not be able to stand the strain, and physical damage will occur. In many cases the weakest component turns out to be the flexor tendons, and they show varying degrees of physical breakdown. The severity of the injury can vary enormously, from a slight bowing of the tendon to complete rupture of one of the flexor tendons. The pathological changes which take place vary only in severity. The changes in a bowed tendon, where the horse is still basically sound, are the same as those in a 'broken-down' horse which has a grossly swollen leg that it is unwilling to put any weight on at all.

Tendon injuries
Tendons tend to suffer sprains at certain specific points along their length. Fig 11 shows these common sites. Some authorities hold that the flexor tendons are more likely to be injured in the mid-cannon region because the blood supply to the core of the tendon in this region is very poor. This explanation does not apply, however, to the other common sites of sprain and it is perhaps more likely that physical factors of leverage, conformation and gait are more important in determining where and when a tendon is going to give way.

When we look at the physical forces which are acting on the flexor ten-

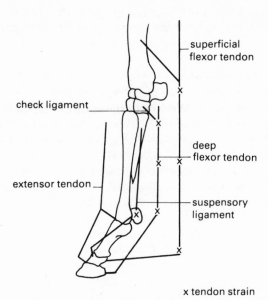

x tendon strain

Fig 11 Common sites of tendon strains

dons of a perfectly normal horse, it has been calculated that the tendons have a tensile strength of 5-10kg/mm². As the cross-sectional area at their narrowest point is around 500mm² the maximum force which they could be asked to transmit safely would be 25-50,000N (N is a unit of force equivalent to 1kg/m/sec².) Now a galloping Thoroughbred is reckoned to be generating a force of about 11,000N on its single weight-bearing foot just before it enters the suspension phase of the gait, and the fulcrum effect of the angle of the fetlock joint increases this two- or threefold to 22-33,000N. The healthy flexor tendon is thus operating well within its potential danger limits even in normal situations. Given the fatigue levels at which it is so often asked to perform, and the uneven surfaces on which it is so often asked to perform, it is really a wonder that any athletic horse manages to avoid tendon strain at all.

As sprains of the flexor tendons are possibly the commonest soft-tissue injury suffered by the athletic horse, and are certainly responsible for more time lost from the training schedule than any other, it is important to understand in some detail the microscopic changes which are occurring in order to be able to look at treatments and alterations in the training programme objectively rather than subjectively as is so often the case at the moment. Although we know the unfavourable changes

which can occur during exercise, we cannot as yet describe any beneficial effects of training on the microscopic structure of tendons. Everyone
accepts that slow work 'hardens' tendons, but nobody has seen this for
themselves under the microscope. Just as there has been a dearth of
factual scientific data available on such changes in the normal anatomy
of tendons, until the publication of the so-called 'Silver Report' in 1983,
there was relatively little known about the pathology of tendon injuries.

The healthy tendon has parallel collagen fibres lying in a background
matrix which contains very few cells. The collagen fibrils are waved and
crimped in a regular pattern, and it is this crimping which allows the
normal stretching of the tendon when under strain. Anything which
alters the crimping will also alter the ability of the tendon to react to
normal load forces. Collagen is a common structural protein in the body,
and there are slightly different types of collagen used for differing purposes. Healthy tendon has Type I collagen in the tendon itself with
Types III, IV and V collagen in the tissues around the tendon. These collagen types are important because, whereas Type I collagen has good
tensile strength, a very desirable attribute in a tendon, Types III, IV and
V are associated far more with elasticity, which is not quite the same
thing and nowhere near as desirable.

The first sign that there is a problem with a tendon is usually the
development of some heat and swelling around the tendon. At this stage
the actual tendon may not be swollen at all, it is just the tendon sheath
which appears to be affected. This warning sign should not be ignored,
however, because if it were possible to look into the tendon with a microscope we would already see evidence of damage. The reason why we first
see changes in the tissues around the tendon is because it is from these
tissues that the first inflammatory cells migrate into the tendon itself.
This reaction is also responsible for the first long-term effect of tendon
sprain, because the movement of these cells and the accumulation of
inflammatory tissue fluid around the tendon will often give rise to
adhesions between the tendon sheath and the tendon. These adhesions
will, of course, limit normal movement of the tendon within the sheath
during exercise.

The area of damaged tendon becomes changed from the structure we
described earlier with very few cells to a very cellular substance. The
horse's body manufactures granulation tissue, which is its standard response to damage whether it is a skin wound or a strained tendon. The
increased number of cells and the new fibres which are laid down cause a
marked thickening of the tendon. The cross-sectional area may be increased to three or four times the normal. You must not equate this increase in size with any increase in strength, however. The exact opposite

is the case; the tendon is at its weakest at this stage. Microscopic examination of this damaged tendon shows that there are areas of necrotic or
dead tissue inside the tendon. One of the reasons for the tendon dying
within these areas is that the tearing of the collagen fibres which occurs
in a strained tendon damages the tiny arteries which feed the normal
tendon, and without this blood supply the tendon tissue will die. Contrary to popular opinion, a sprained tendon has an excellent blood
supply.

The granulation tissue which is formed at the site of a tendon sprain
soon starts to make new collagen fibres as it starts to rebuild the more
normal structure of the tendon. Unfortunately, the fibres which are
made do not lie in parallel bundles along the direction of maximum pull
on the tendon, as they normally do. Instead, they have a very irregular
pattern. Initially, they have no crimp at all, and so no ability to extend
in response to the strain of work. Even when eventually fibres with a
crimp pattern are laid down, it is not the normal pattern. The normal
pattern will still not have been returned to as long as fourteen months
after the horse first sprained the tendon. Nor is the collagen in these
fibres the collagen Type I which it needs to be for maximum tensile
strength. Instead, it is Type III, IV and V collagen. Measurements have
shown that up to 30 per cent of a damaged tendon may be Type III collagen. Examinations of damaged tendons have again shown that even
fourteen months after the injury, some of this Type III collagen will remain, weakening the apparently healed tendon.

Horse owners have observed for centuries that if a horse sprains a tendon on one leg, it will often strain the tendon on the leg on the opposite
side at a later date. In many cases this second injury occurs just as the
horse has returned to maximum performance after treatment for the
initial strain. It was thought that this second injury occurred because
there was a basic weakness in both tendons which was bound to result in
both of them becoming strained as a result of the strain of work. Many
veterinary surgeons have recommended accordingly that when a horse
suffers a strained tendon, the corresponding tendon on the other leg
should be treated at the same time, as a preventive measure.

We now know that this is not exactly what is happening. If we look at
that other leg at the time of the original injury, we see that it is usually
completely normal. Over the following weeks and months, however,
very marked changes occur. These are thought to be the result of the
extra weight which this tendon has to support twenty-four hours a day
because the 'bad' leg is too weak and painful to share the weight equally.
What happens is that the 'good' tendon also starts to manufacture Type
III collagen and the normal crimp pattern is lost. These hidden changes

are at their most marked around nine months after the original injury, just at the time when the horse may well appear completely sound and be back in work again.

The problem of repeated tendon sprains of the same leg was thought to be due to a basic fault in the tendon such as a particularly poor blood supply. The work on healing tendons carried out by Professor Silver at Bristol University shows that it is far more a problem that the microscopic structure of the tendon takes much longer to return to normal than does the gross anatomy. The horse is thus returned to work on the basis of visible soundness despite invisible weaknesses. In many cases, the horse manages to cope with the situation and remains sound even during the initial six or nine months of further healing, but in other cases the weakened tendon gives way again. It is thought that the persistent presence of inflammatory fluids between the collagen fibrils in such partially healed tendons is largely responsible for their weakness. Another factor is that even when the horse appears sound to an experienced observer, there may still be alterations in its gait. High-speed film of such horses has shown that the injured leg is not placed flatly on the ground, with the sole of the foot parallel to the ground. Instead, the toe hits the ground first, and even when the leg is completely weight-bearing, the fetlock angle is markedly more upright than normal. As we have discussed earlier, this will have a marked effect on the forces which have to be borne by all parts of that leg, and some part of the system may give way again.

The final piece of equine folklore about healing tendons is that the repaired portion of the tendon is stronger than the original, and that is why any further strain will tend to occur just above or just below the original injury. As we have seen, the granulation tissue of a healing tendon certainly does not have as high a tensile strength as the healthy tendon because the Type III collagen actually has less tensile strength than the original Type I collagen. The area of granulation tissue is, however, rather like a mass of tangled wool with fibres interwoven in all directions rather than in parallel rows. It is, therefore, relatively difficult to pull this mass apart by pulling on its top and bottom. If the force is too great, it is more likely to cause tearing at the points where the undamaged tendon merges into the granulation tissue, and this give a new injury just above or just below the original. It is rather like a piece of furniture – the joints are always the weakest spots.

The treatment of strained tendons

As tendon strain is such an important injury of the athletic horse, both in terms of its high incidence rate and of the disruption of training schedules which it causes, every trainer should be au fait with the various treatment regimes and understand how they are supposed to work. The very variety of these treatments should warn us straight away that there is no guaranteed, rapid cure for strained tendons. When rapid cures do apparently occur, it is most likely that the problem lay more in the tendon sheath than in the body of the tendon itself. These sheaths completely surround the tendons, and when the tendon moves during exercise, it does so within a stationary tendon sheath. The inner surface of the sheath and the outer surface of the tendon are both smooth, so that there is as little friction as possible between them. Friction is further reduced by the presence of a small amount of lubricating fluid. It is possible to have a bowed, or swollen, tendon where the vast majority of the symptoms of inflammation, ie the heat, swelling, pain and oedema, are associated with the tendon sheath rather than the tendon. As the sheath is only a relatively few cells thick and has a good blood supply, it can heal quickly. Indeed, it is desirable that it should do so because if it remains inflamed, there is the possibility that adhesions may form across the gap between sheath and tendon. So, a damaged tendon sheath may repair itself in weeks, but a strained tendon will take months to heal.

A strained tendon is an inflamed tendon above all else. Inflammation is usually associated with the accumulation of inflammatory fluids brought to the area by an increased blood supply. The first basic treatment is the application of a cold compress. This causes the blood-vessels to constrict and so reduces the numbers of inflammatory cells, etc which are moved into the area. There are numerous sources of cold available, including cold-water bandages, ice-packs, chemical cooling packs and substances such as kaolin which are cooled down in a refrigerator and will then hold their heat for a long time. A long time is, however, relative and it is surprising how quickly a cold compress is warmed up by the heat of an acutely strained tendon. The sooner you can apply support and cold to a strained tendon the better it is. Thankfully, the practice of applying a hot poultice to these tendons has more or less died out. It increases the blood supply at exactly the wrong moment and so tends to increase swelling rather than decrease it. Whatever treatment is subsequently to be used, cold compresses should always be the initial treatment. They should be started as soon as possible and continued until the heat and pain of the strain have subsided.

The next stage of recovery will not be hurried by artificial means, and there are many authorities which consider that rest alone is all that is required to obtain a good resolution of a strained tendon. The period of rest which is necessary will depend to a great extent on the severity of the strain itself, and it is not, unfortunately, possible to lay down hard guidelines. In the case of an acute strain, a period of at least nine months' rest will be necessary before the tendon achieves both visible and functional normality. Microscopically, of course, repair will still not have been completed within nine months. Rest does not imply that the horse should be confined to its stable and never come out. Nor does it mean that the horse should be turned out in a field and allowed to walk or gallop about at will. It has been found that the best course is to confine the horse to its stable but to give it one or two periods of walking out in hand every day. Initially, each period should only last about ten minutes but in the later stages this may be increased. When considering the relative effectiveness of other methods of treatment, we must assess them against what can be achieved by rest alone.

Firing

For the past couple of hundred years controversy has raged over the effectiveness or otherwise of 'firing' as a method of treatment for strained tendons. This involves the use of a red-hot iron to cause a regulated burn over the strained area on the grounds that the inflammation so induced will also speed up healing of the tendon strain. The iron is either used to make parallel lines almost, but not quite, through the whole skin thickness, or a pointed iron is used to make incisions through the skin into the body of the tendon. These methods are called line and pin firing respectively. The hope is that firing will produce a supportive 'bandage' of thickened, scarred skin which will support the damaged tendon. At the same time it is hoped to speed up the healing process by increasing the blood supply to the area and causing a healed scar to look more like the original tendon. Firing is not carried out until the initial inflammatory period is over.

The 'Silver Report' was the result of research carried out at the University of Bristol following questions in the House of Commons about the welfare aspects of firing. It looked at firing on a scientific basis for the very first time, and was unable to support the claims made for it as a means of treatment. Professor Silver found that, far from thickening the skin to give support, firing causes a thinning of the skin when the affected area is examined under a microscope. As part of the horse's reaction to the firing, a large amount of inflammatory fluid accumulates around the tendon and this causes adhesions onto the tendon which are inhibitory rather than useful. Line firing does not result in any permanent change in the structure of the tendon itself, but pin firing does leave scars of dense collagen along the track of the firing iron. Firing does not appear to affect the amount of Type III collagen which is formed for better or for worse.

Professor Silver did find some adverse effects from firing. The links which normally form between the crimped fibrils of collagen in normal tendons are much slower to reappear after firing than they are in horses which have just been rested. Horses which are fired appear to develop more marked changes in the other leg than would otherwise be the case. The report stated that some fired animals became indistinguishable from those which were untreated after about six months but then deteriorated in relation to the untreated animal during the following three months and finally returned to the normal recovery pattern in a further three months.

Tendon-splitting and carbon-fibre operations

During the 1960s Swedish workers pioneered a surgical treatment for strained tendons, the so-called tendon-splitting operation. Originally, this involved making a long vertical incision through the skin into the body of the flexor tendon. The outer layers were then stitched up but the tendon was allowed to heal in its own time. The operation is now more commonly carried out by making a series of stab incisions through the skin with a stiletto-type knife and then moving the blade of the knife through an arc so that the cut into the tendon is much longer than that through the skin. A series of these incisions are made starting just above the injured part of the tendon and extending right through it into the normal tendon again. The rationale behind the operation is that the incisions into the belly of the tendon provide an easy pathway for new blood-vessels to follow into the damaged area. Once there, these blood-vessels are expected to result in quicker and better healing.

Having shown that, even from the earliest days, a damaged tendon had a much increased blood supply right into the depths of the tendon, Professor Silver's team felt that any method which simply aimed at increasing the blood supply would be ineffective in speeding up tendon healing. Horses which had had a tendon-splitting operation were observed as they trotted over a force plate and it was found that they took significantly longer to return to normal function than horses which had merely been rested.

Professor Silver's final conclusions were that 'On the basis of our pathological investigation, we can find no evidence that line firing or pin firing of the skin has any marked effect on tendon healing although in one or two cases it appeared to delay the process. Tendon splitting, on the other hand, was *clearly* deleterious and pin firing into the tendon *appeared* to be. None of these procedures hastened normal healing, or improved its quality, with the possible exception of the provision of a correctly aligned artificial scaffold such as carbon fibre.' These conclusions have aroused a great deal of controversy in the UK. Veterinary surgeons who routinely fire large numbers of horses remain convinced that, no matter what the microscope may say, fired horses withstand the stresses of further training better than those which have just been rested. Unfortunately, no statistical evidence has yet been put forward to support this view. There is evidence that horses which have had a tendon-splitting operation can have as much success on the trotting track as normal horses, but there is no evidence to show that these successes are greater than those achieved by horses which have simply been given adequate rest.

Paradoxically, the tendon-splitting operation, which Professor Silver found to be ineffective, has led the way to the most promising new surgical technique. This is the use of a prosthesis, an artificial replacement for part of the natural body, in the healing tendon. The operation is basically the same as the original tendon-splitting operation which was described earlier, but when the tendon has been split open a bundle of artificial fibres is laid along the cut before everything is stitched up again. At the time of writing, the most popular material to use is a row of carbon fibres. These are not used for any tensile strength; indeed, the surgical technique does not anchor them firmly enough for this to be achieved. Instead, they are used to provide a scaffolding along which fibroblasts and collagen fibres can grow. Carbon filaments are ideal for this purpose because they are so smooth and have such a regular diameter. By encouraging the collagen fibres to grow along straight lines which are in the direction of stress in the tendon, a repair is obtained which is more like the original structure. These carbon fibres, incidentally, are not removed but are left in place, carbon being a very inactive substance which does not stimulate a rejection response from the tendon. Carbon fibres are not the ideal prosthesis, however, and the search is now on for better substances to use. In particular, a substance is being sought which will encourage the development of a more natural crimp pattern than occurs with carbon fibres.

Other treatments
Some practitioners use a technique called acid firing in the treatment of sprained tendons. This involves applying dilute acid to the skin over the tendon, using a mask to restrict it to small circular areas rather like the pattern used in pin firing. The effect of this must be rather similar to the age-old practice of blistering the leg, although more severe. Blistering is

the application of an irritant substance, often a mercuric iodide, to the skin. It causes an intense inflammation, with profuse weeping of inflammatory fluid from the blisters which form. The severity of the reaction is dependent on both the amount of chemical used and the length of time spent rubbing it into the skin. The idea behind the treatment is to produce a thickened support for the tendon underneath the skin. So far, no work has been carried out to see exactly what effect blistering has on tendon healing, but at first sight it appears unlikely that it will be in any way different from the effect of line firing.

If the tendon-splitting operation was the fashionable treatment for sprained tendons in the Sixties and Seventies, magnetic therapy is the fashionable treatment of the mid-Eighties. This is probably partly due to the fact that horse owners can embark on this therapy without any recourse to their veterinary surgeon, and they like to feel that they can diagnose and treat their horse's ailments. This has led to problems in assessing the efficacy of the treatments because if an owner has instituted the treatment, he wants to believe that it has been successful. Surveys of horses which have received magnetic therapy show that the owners usually think that it has had more effect than independent scientific observers looking at the same horse before and after treatment!

Magnetic therapy is the placing of a magnetic field around the injured area. This might be done using permanent magnets incorporated in a material which is wrapped around the tendon, or it might involve the

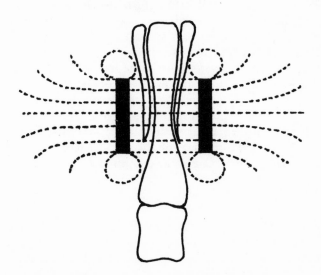

Fig 12 Diagram of electromagnetic field induced in horse's cannon

use of a pulsing electro-magnetic field, induced using parallel coils (Fig 12). Pulsing electro-magnetic therapy has been proved to be effective in speeding up the healing of certain fractures in human beings and evidence is now becoming available that it is also effective in some shoulder injuries. There is, as yet, no scientific evidence that magnetic therapy can speed up or improve the quality of healing of sprained tendons. It would not be wise, however, to rule this out completely. The application of electro-magnetic fields to such tendons certainly does sometimes produce some sort of reaction, as shown by the development of heat and swelling around the area and, as previously mentioned, some horse owners feel it is very beneficial. It is difficult for the veterinary profession to get very excited over a therapy when we have no idea how it works (despite the vague statements to the contrary made in much of the advertising for this equipment). At the present time it appears likely that magnetic fields can alter the electro-chemical information on the individual cell membrane, but how this speeds up the repair of sprained tendons is not known.

What, then, is the horse owner to do when faced with a sprained tendon? First of all, the time for seeking veterinary advice is immediately after it happens, not days or weeks later. It may be possible to use anti-inflammatory drugs to limit the initial inflammatory response. Anything which reduces the amount of inflammatory fluid which accumulates is to the good, so keep the leg cold. Laser therapy, which will be discussed in Chapter 4, may be of value. Once the initial inflammation has subsided, the horse should be walked out for a short time daily so that the normal tension forces on the tendon can stimulate the collagen fibres to be laid down in a uniform rather than haphazard way. The amount of rest which will be necessary will depend on the severity of the injury, but remember that normal microscopic structure will not be regained for several months after the horse becomes sound again. This warning is especially appropriate when laser therapy has produced a very rapid and complete improvement in symptoms. On balance, a period of at least a year's rest is probably the best treatment which can be recommended on scientific grounds for an acutely sprained tendon.

Plate 4 X-ray of a horse's foot showing navicular disease. The arrows indicate the rough and eroded surface of the navicular bone

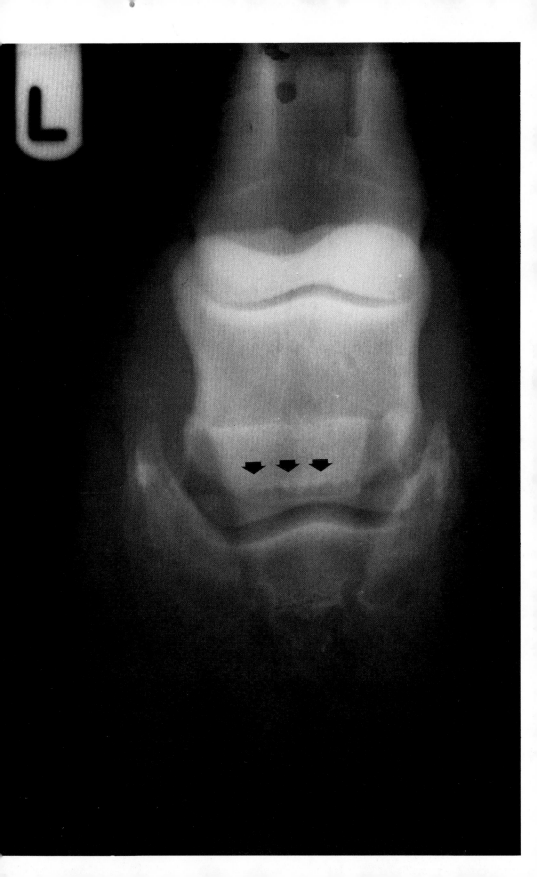

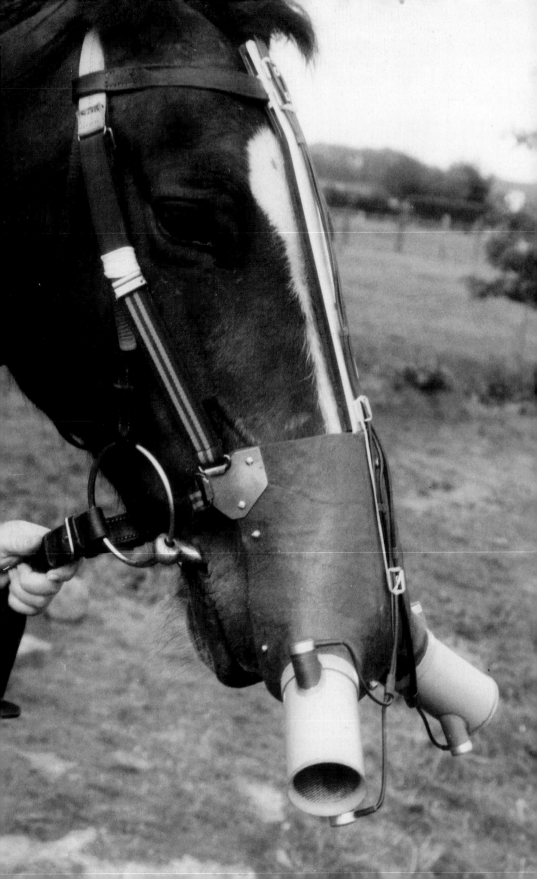

3 · Understanding Energy and its Relationship to Performance

Within the universe energy exists in a number of different forms, as light, chemical, heat, electrical and mechanical energy. Life can only continue because living organisms, from the simplest to the most complicated, can convert energy from one form to another. With the exception of the very simplest of processes, such as the passage of small molecules across the cell membranes, most of the processes which make up a biological system require the use of chemical energy. Most of this chemical energy is formed during a complex sequence of reactions during which fuels are broken down and chemical energy released. During the various metabolic processes which make up the biological system which we call life, chemical energy is converted into heat energy or vice versa. In the case of movement, some of the chemical energy has also first to be converted into mechanical as well as heat energy. As shown in Fig 13, this energy release can be compared to the way that mechanical energy is taken from water in a hydro-electric plant.

The amount of energy used or produced in a process is measured in a unit called a joule (J). In scientific circles, this has now replaced the older form of measurement, the calorie (cal). Most horse owners will be familiar with the calorie for the wrong reasons. Its use in the world of slimming diets, etc has caused it to be thought of as simply a measure of how fattening a particular foodstuff is. As we shall see, energy is produced in many more situations than simply during the digestion of food. One calorie is equal to 4.2J, and it is defined as the amount of energy necessary to raise the temperature of 1g of water by 1.8°F (1°C). One kilocalorie (kcal) or 1 kilojoule (kJ) are one thousand times a calorie or joule respectively.

When considering movement, or locomotion, the amount of work performed is roughly equivalent to the amount of energy expended. The term 'work' simply implies that the energy has, in this case, been used to

Plate 5 Mask system for measuring respiratory flow rates and oxygen consumption (*courtesy A. Woakes*)

move a mass over a certain distance. A study of elementary physics shows that:

Work = Force × distance moved

For practical purposes on flat ground:

Work performed = Horse's weight × distance moved

Power (P) refers to the amount of work or energy expended per unit of time, so when we refer to power there is always a concept of time in-

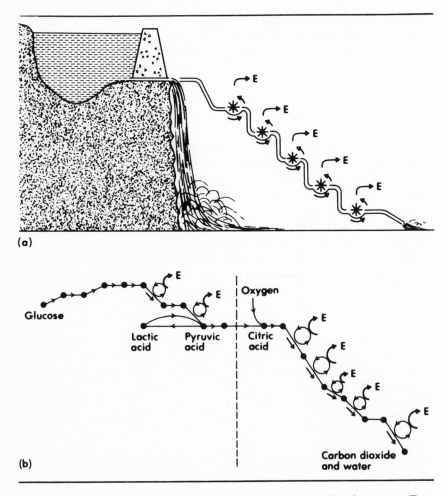

(a)

(b)

Fig 13 Energy during metabolism is released in a similar way to that from water (From *Physical Fitness and Athletic Performance*, A.W.S. Watson, Longman, London, 1983)

volved. As a result, the greater the speed at which the horse travels, the higher its power output. It is the maximal power output that is important, for example, in sprinting events. As we shall see, the maximum power output of a Quarterhorse will be considerably greater than that possible in an endurance horse.

How the horse obtains its energy

Within the cells of the horse's body, the immediate source of chemical energy for processes such as locomotion, is a compound called adenosine triphosphate (ATP) (Fig 14). The important part of this complicated name is *tri*phosphate, because the energy which is stored within this molecule is stored in the three phosphate bonds. When each of these three phosphate particles is broken off, a small quantity of energy is released. Usually, only one of the phosphate particles is broken off. The reaction needs the presence of a special catalyst, or enzyme, and water.

$$ATP + H_2O \longrightarrow (enzyme) \longrightarrow ADP + P + Energy$$

When energy is being used for movement, only part of the energy that is produced will be mechanical energy. The rest will be lost as heat. So, only about 25 per cent of the energy is actually used to produce movement, which is not a very high level of efficiency. As a result, large numbers of molecules of ATP have to be broken down to ADP during any kind of movement. During sprinting in man, for example, it has been calculated that each stride requires the breakdown of ten to the power twenty (which is more than a billion billion) molecules of ATP.

The amount of ATP stored within cells is extremely limited, and it has been calculated that there is only sufficient inside a muscle cell to provide the energy for two or three muscle cell contractions. So muscular work cannot be maintained unless further supplies of ATP are provided (Fig 14). In fact, the horse does not make new ATP, but rather it recycles the old ADP molecule. This reverses the initial reaction:

$$ADP + P + Energy \longrightarrow (enzyme) \longrightarrow ATP + H_2O$$

The rate at which the ATP is reformed obviously needs to keep pace with the rate at which the original amount of ATP within the muscle cell is broken down to provide energy. The faster the horse is moving, the more rapid the regeneration of ATP needs to be.

The horse obviously needs a source of energy to add to the ADP and the phosphate in order to resynthesise the ATP. For this it uses chemical energy which it obtains from certain substances within the body. These chemical energy stores come from the horse's food. Now food consists of a

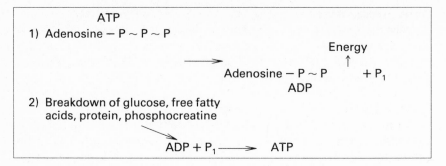

Fig 14 1) Energy is provided when the molecule ATP consisting of adenosine plus 3 phosphate groups has the terminal phosphate broken off, this then allows biological work to be performed. 2) Reformation of ADP to ATP occurs when simple compounds from foods are broken down to release energy that can be stored by reattaching the third phosphate group to ADP.

mixture of substances, including carbohydrates, fats and proteins. All three of these food constituents contain chemical energy which can be released when the food is broken down. The two major sources of energy are carbohydrates and fats. Except during starvation, proteins are of little importance as energy sources. As long as oxygen is present, both carbohydrates and fats can be completely broken down. The resulting carbon dioxide and water contain much less chemical energy than the original fuel because much of that energy has been released for the horse's use. It is sometimes convenient to speak of oxygen being used to 'burn' a fuel in order to produce energy. If a litre of oxygen is used up to burn either carbohydrate or fat, it will release about 20kJ (5kcal) of energy.

Storing energy for future use
When a horse needs to store carbohydrate within its body so that it will have a future source of energy, it does so as a compound called glycogen. This consists of thousands of glucose molecules formed into a single branched molecule (Fig 15). Large numbers of these glucose molecules can then be broken off the glycogen molecule when they are needed for energy production. Glycogen is stored in the horse's liver and in its muscle cells. Wherever you find it, you always also find the enzymes needed for its synthesis and breakdown. The stores of glycogen in the liver are used to supply glucose for all the tissues of the body, including nerves, blood cells, etc. There is a constant release of glucose from the glycogen of the liver into the blood in order to meet these tissue requirements. The body needs to be able to rely on a set level of glucose in the blood, and so there is a sophisticated system of hormones which controls the amount of glucose released from the liver in order to maintain this

blood-glucose level even at times of high demand from the body. The glycogen which is stored in the muscles, on the other hand, is not available to the other body tissues; it is only broken down when its glucose is required by the muscle itself. The new glycogen which is required to maintain these energy stores, which is what the two glycogen stores are, is built up from glucose and other substances derived from the absorption and breakdown of carbohydrates from the horse's diet.

Fat is the other major fuel store. It is composed of triglyceride molecules. Each of these has one molecule of glycerol to which three molecules of fatty acids are attached. Some of these triglyceride molecules are stored within cells throughout the body, including muscle cells. There are also collections of more specialised cells which store triglycerides in adipose tissue. This adipose tissue is the 'fat' which we human beings spend so much time, effort, and money trying to eliminate from our bodies. It is the fat layer beneath the skin, around major organs such as the heart, and in the abdominal cavity. The amount of adipose tissue present in each horse varies widely, although it is obviously greater in a 'fat' horse.

There is more than thirty times the amount of energy stored within a horse's adipose tissue than there is in all the glycogen within its body. Even a lean horse will have enough fat available to enable it to exercise at a moderate pace for several days. However, as will be discussed later,

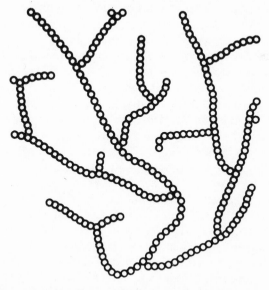

Fig 15 A glycogen molecule consists of a large number of glucose molecules
(The Runner, E. Newsholme & T. Leech, Fitness Books, New Jersey.)

it is not actually possible to maintain moderate speeds solely burning fat. There is, therefore, no point in a horse carrying excess fat when it is competing in endurance rides. In fact, a fat horse is at a disadvantage in two ways. First, excess fat means that more energy has to be used up in moving the extra weight of horse around. Secondly, the insulating properties of the fat reduce heat loss from the horse, which can have far-reaching consequences.

How the various fuels are utilised

Now that we have discussed how the fuels are stored, we can consider how and when they are used. During most types of equestrian exercise, it is necessary to use both kinds of stored energy. In the case of glycogen, glucose molecules are split off as a result of enzyme action. The glycogen in the muscles is, of course, immediately available, but that in the liver has to be transported first via the bloodstream to the muscles which are working at any particular moment. Triglycerides are broken down in order to release their fatty acids into the blood. These fatty acids are not transported just as they are, however, but have first to be fastened onto a protein called albumen. They then hitch a lift, as it were, on the albumen to the working muscles where they are needed. The rate at which fatty acids can be taken up by muscles from the blood is limited, and this is one of the reasons why fatty acids cannot be the sole fuel source during exercise. Training increases the amount of free fatty acids that can be used. In some of the muscle cells, triglycerides are also actually broken down to free fatty acids at the 'scene of the action'.

Once within the muscle cell, both glucose and fatty acids pass through a complex chain of reactions that end up in their being reduced to carbon dioxide and water. The initial stages of this chain are carried out in the absence of oxygen, but the final stages can only occur if oxygen is present. These important final stages take place within structures inside the muscle cell which are called the mitochondria. Because almost all the energy is released within these mitochondria, they are often considered to be the powerhouses of the cells. As this kind of energy-producing pathway requires oxygen, it is called aerobic metabolism or oxidative metabolism.

The number of ADP molecules which can be reformed into ATP as a result of the breakdown of one molecule of glucose is 39. One molecule of free fatty acid, on the other hand, will yield 138 molecules of ATP. On a weight basis, 1g of triglyceride gives just over twice as much energy as 1g of glycogen, and so is a much more efficient method of storing energy. Its advantage is further increased by the fact that in storing 1g of glycogen, nearly 3g of water are also trapped in the system. This may have been some advantage in the wild state where fuel supplies varied from day to day, but it is of little relevance today when horses are fed several times a day. Despite all of this, it should be appreciated that both the processes are only about 50 per cent efficient in terms of providing energy which actually regenerates ATP. The rest of the energy is released as heat energy which, during exercise, has to be removed from the body.

Although in most circumstances the energy supplies of the cell can be met by the complete combustion of free fatty acids and glucose, there are situations in which an energy deficit would occur if these were the only ways in which the horse could obtain energy. This means that the horse is undergoing exercise which is so strenuous that it requires more energy than can be provided by normal aerobic metabolism. Such a situation can obviously not exist for any appreciable length of time. To cope with such an eventuality, a system has evolved for rebuilding ATP molecules without using any oxygen. These processes are referred to as anaerobic metabolism.

Stored within the cells is a compound which is classed as a high-energy phosphate. It is called creatine phosphate (CP). In the presence of suitable enzymes, this CP can combine with ADP to recreate ATP.

$$CP + ADP \xrightarrow{\text{enzyme}} ATP + creatine$$

In other words, the high-energy phosphate or the creatine phosphate is passed onto the adenosine diphosphate. There are, of course, only limited amounts of creatine phosphate within the cells, and this will only provide enough energy (via ATP production) for about six to eight seconds of maximal exercise. It would appear that neither feeding nor training can increase the amount of CP stored in the cells. When this super phosphate is used during exercise, it is naturally replaced as soon as sufficient oxygen becomes available to combine with all the ADP and convert it to ATP in the more 'usual' aerobic way. Creatine phosphate is an important source of energy in the early stages of high-intensity exercise, eg acceleration out of the starting gates or jumping. This is especially so because oxygen delivery to the tissues has not reached a very high level in the initial stages of exercise.

There is another very important means of providing ATP when there is a shortage of oxygen. This is by the partial breakdown of glucose. In this reaction, glucose is broken down to lactate and ATP:

$$Glucose \longrightarrow 2\ lactate + 3\ ATP$$

This is obviously a much less efficient way of using glucose than that which has already been discussed. It also has the important disadvantage that lactate is formed which can have a very serious effect on future performance. This is because the lactate, or lactic acid, produced cannot be removed from the cells as fast as it is produced. It then acts like any other acid and decreases the pH of the cell when it builds up over a certain level. When the cell becomes too acid, interference occurs in its normal processes so that its ability to produce further ATP is markedly decreased. The ability of the contractile proteins in the muscles to contract efficiently is also impaired. These processes thus lead to the muscle cell no longer being able to function properly and, as will be discussed later, fatigue sets in. So lactate production cannot be considered as a continuous source of energy.

Part of the effect of the build-up in lactic acid levels is counteracted by the buffering capacity of certain compounds in the muscle. This means that such compounds are relatively alkaline, and neutralise some of the acidic effects which would otherwise occur. At the present time there is some debate as to whether one of the favourable effects of training is to produce an increase in the buffering capacity of muscle cells, and thus to increase the ability of the cell to withstand lactic acid production. As the lactate produced in a cell cannot be utilised by that muscle cell, it passes into the bloodstream. It is then further broken down by other tissues in the body both during and after the exercise being undertaken. This further breakdown of lactate also needs oxygen, and this is why horses still have an increased heart and respiratory rate even after strenuous exercise is completed. They require extra oxygen to remove the excess lactate. As will be discussed later, the rate of removal of the lactate can be influenced by the work done during this recovery period.

Table 1 Average fuels available for energy generation in a 450kg horse

Fuel	Tissue	Grams
Glycogen	Liver	150
Glycogen	Muscle	3,600
Triglyceride	Adipose	40,000
Triglyceride	Muscle	2,000
Protein	Muscle	38,000

The amounts of the differing fuels which are available for ATP formation are summarised in Table 1. In Fig 16 the relative advantages and disadvantages of fat and carbohydrate as fuels are listed.

Adapting the energy source to the type of work being performed
When a horse is working, it does not simply use one energy source at a time. The relative amounts of the different sources used for the regeneration of ATP depends on factors such as the severity of the exercise, its

duration and the fitness of the horse. During rest, muscle uses free fatty acids to provide the energy for keeping the powerhouse 'ticking over'. As the muscles start to work, glucose is also used. The more the horse works, the higher the percentage of glucose that is being used as the energy source, until at fast work glucose is the major energy source. This change-over of the principal energy source from free fatty acid to glucose occurs partly because the rapidly contracting muscle cells cannot obtain sufficient fatty acid, and partly because glucose is more efficient in terms of the use it makes of any available oxygen. Having said this, at slow speeds, such as the walk and trot, the longer the exercise lasts, the higher the proportion of free fatty acids which will be used (Fig 16). The proportion of free fatty acids used at any speed is higher in fit horses. One of the effects of training is to increase the amount of the enzymes responsible for the uptake and breakdown of this fuel. The advantage of this is that it leads to what is called a glycogen sparing effect, and this is important when considering the causes of fatigue.

At light work almost all the energy needed can be obtained from aerobic metabolism, with just a very small amount from the partial breakdown of glucose to lactate. Because only small amounts of lactate are being produced, they are quickly removed from around the cells by

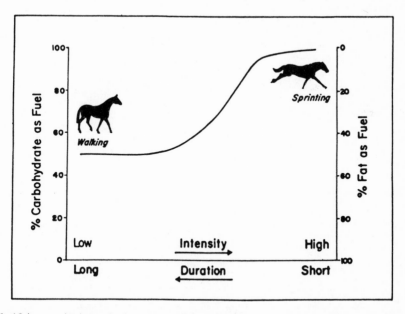

Fig 16 As exercise intensity increases and duration decreases, the predominant food fuel is carbohydrate. (Adapted from *Sports Physiology,* E.L. Fox, 2nd edition. Saunders College Publishing, New York)

the general blood circulation and taken away to be safely broken down. However, at a certain speed or severity of work (which varies according to the fitness of that particular horse), the situation is reached where insufficient energy can be obtained from aerobic methods. In a reasonably fit horse this point is reached when it is moving at around 656yd (600m) per minute. Although traditionally this situation has been thought to have occurred because of a lack of oxygen, the real reasons are still not generally agreed. The important point is that the increased energy demands can only be met by also obtaining part of the energy requirements from anaerobic metabolism. As a result, the faster the horse works, the higher the percentage of the energy which comes from lactate

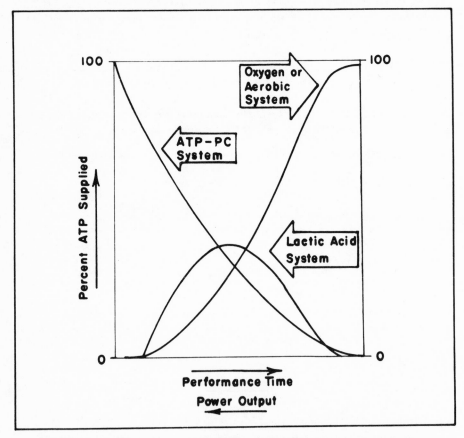

Fig 17 The relationship between percent ATP contributed by the three energy systems as related to performance time or power output. The shorter the performance time, the greater the output and the more rapid the energy (ATP) requirement. (Adapted from *Sports Physiology*, E.L. Fox, 2nd edition. Saunders College Publishing, New York)

production. The lactate passes into the blood, and this is the reason why ever-increasing amounts of lactate are seen in the blood as the horse goes faster. As well as burning glucose to lactate, the energy supply is also topped up in the initial stages by the breakdown of creatine phosphate.

Anaerobic metabolism is not only important as the horse moves faster and faster. It is also extremely important during explosive movements, such as accelerating out of starting gates or in jumping. The contribution aerobic and anaerobic metabolisms make to the various activities in men and horses is shown in Fig 17 and Table 2.

Table 2 Estimated energy contributed in man from aerobic and anaerobic metabolism when running at maximum speed for varying times

Time	Aerobic %	Anaerobic %
10 sec	15	85
1 min	30-35	65-70
2 min	50	50
4 min	70	30
10 min	80-85	10-15
30 min	95	5
60 min	98	2
120 min	99	1

Meeting oxygen requirements during energy production

The ability to produce energy by aerobic metabolism is obviously dependent on the amount of oxygen that can be utilised by the mitochondia which form the powerhouses of the cells. It is also dependent on sufficient oxygen being delivered to the muscles in the first place. As the oxygen coming into the system originates in the air which the horse breathes in, there are a number of factors which can influence this supply and they can be summarised as follows:

1 Lung ventilation.
2 The passage of oxygen from the lungs into the blood.
3 The rate at which the oxygen is transported around the circulation. This in turn depends on the output of the heart and the oxygen-carrying capacity of the blood.
4 The passage of oxygen from the blood out into the muscle.

These factors will be discussed in later chapters.

The amount of oxygen which is used by the body is referred to as its oxygen uptake or consumption. It is usually measured as the number of millilitres of oxygen consumed per kilogram of body-weight per minute. Oxygen consumption is usually abbreviated to VO_2, and the maximum amount that can be utilised is called VO_2 max. The VO_2 max would appear to be determined genetically as well as by training. When a horse exercises, the amount of oxygen it consumes increases in a straight line as it does more and more work. Eventually, a plateau is reached when oxygen consumption no longer increases although the horse may increase its workload (Fig 18). In fact, the increase in oxygen

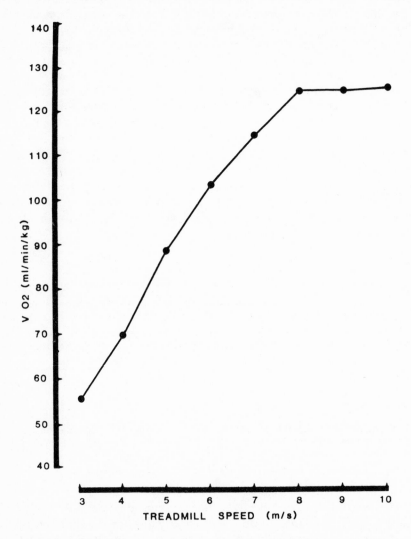

Fig 18 The relationship of oxygen consumption to workload. Note the plateauing of oxygen consumption at higher speeds. Results obtained from horses working on a treadmill at an incline. (Courtesy D. Evans and R. Rose).

consumption closely parallels the rise in heart rate which takes place. In man, oxygen consumption can increase by about twenty-fold during exercise, and in elite athletes a VO_2 max of about 80ml/kg/min would not be unusual. As an illustration of the degree of adaptation for exercise which is possible in the horse, it has been found that the VO_2 max may be of the order of 140 ml/kg/min. This represents the consumption of about 63 litres of oxygen by a 990lb (450kg) horse, and is a thirty-five-fold increase on resting levels. The horse achieves this higher capacity for aerobic metabolism because of a greater ability to deliver oxygen to the sites which need it. Compared with man, the horse has a greater ability to increase its cardiac output and a greater supply of red blood cells to transport the oxygen.

Oxygen consumption is usually measured by finding out the difference in oxygen levels between the air breathed in and that breathed out. This is then multiplied by the volume of air breathed in and out per minute. In man this measurement is easy to carry out, but in the horse it requires the animal to wear a mask to which are attached tubes to allow collection of the expired air (Plate 5). Athough this is difficult, various methods have been devised to carry out these measurements in the horse, but sometimes problems are still encountered in measuring the consumption at high work rates. Perhaps surprisingly horses tolerate wearing these masks extremely well while exercising on a treadmill or on the track.

The ability to measure oxygen consumption at rest, during work and also during recovery when lactic acid is metabolised and phosphagens restored, allows us to determine accurately the energy cost of the work we have asked the horse to carry out. Obviously, this is very valuable when it comes to devising an effective feeding regime for the horse.

The overall control of energy production
Energy production does not take place in isolation. The increased energy requirements of working muscles require adequate fuel and oxygen supplies before they can take place, and the removal of waste products afterwards. How this is brought about will be discussed in later chapters. However, at this point we should mention how nervous and hormonal activity helps to integrate the whole system.

It is the role of the nervous system within the body to ensure that the body always acts in a co-ordinated way. The nervous system can be looked upon as comprising the central nervous system, ie the brain and spinal cord, and the peripheral nervous system. The latter can, in turn, be broken down into the nerve fibres concerned with sensations of various kinds, such as pain, heat and touch, into the motor nerves which control the voluntary response of skeletal muscles, and into the autonomic or involuntary system. It is the autonomic nervous system which plays such a large regulatory role in controlling the generation and supply of energy. In turn, it is divided into two parts. One part helps in the build-up and conservation of energy, and so largely operates when the horse is at rest. The other part of the autonomic system is called the sympathetic system and is activated during times of stress. When we refer to the horse's adaptation for fright and flight, it is the sympathetic nervous system which takes overall control.

When an impulse passes along a nerve fibre of the sympathetic system (and each individual nerve fibre can be quite long), a substance called nor-adrenalin, or nor-epinephrine, is produced. It is the action of this compound on such organs as the small airways of the lungs, the sweat glands in the skin, the heart and the spleen, that brings about the responses so necessary in stress or life-threatening situations. In the organs just referred to, nor-adrenalin can produce the dilation of airways to allow more oxygen delivery, the initiation of sweating to control body temperature, elevated heart rate to help increase the blood supply to the muscles, and the contraction of the spleen to release more red blood cells into the circulation so that more oxygen can be transported around the body. The sympathetic system also has nerves which go to the adrenal glands, very small organs which lie in front of each kidney. The adrenal gland releases adrenalin, or epinephrine, into the bloodstream. This compound helps in the release of glucose from the liver and in the release of free fatty acids from fat depots. The rise in the blood concentration of adrenalin, and the effects it produces, are very closely related to the intensity of the exercise, ie during endurance events only a small increase in circulating adrenalin occurs, while during racing rises of tenfold or more may take place.

Nor-adrenalin is referred to as a neurotransmitter because it is released from the nerve endings. Adrenalin, on the other hand, is classed as a hormone. A hormone is a substance which is produced in one organ and then transported via the blood to exert its effect elsewhere. A large number of hormones have already been discovered, and new ones are constantly being added to the list. They vary from very small molecules such as adrenalin to very complex proteins such as insulin. They serve numerous functions concerned with maintaining the homeostasis (ie the internal environment) of the body. In addition to adrenalin being important in mobilising fuels for use by the muscles, two other hormones which are produced by a small abdominal organ called the pancreas, glucagon and insulin, are also important in controlling blood-glucose levels. Glucagon is produced when blood-glucose levels are too low, and insulin when the blood glucose is too high. There is also a hormone called cortisol which, like adrenalin, is produced from part of the adrenal gland. We will discuss the role of cortisol in inflammation in a later chapter, but it is important to mention in the present context that it helps in the long-term supply of fuels by increasing the mobilisation of fat, and even in severe circumstances by causing the breakdown of muscle proteins so that they can be metabolised to glucose in the horse's liver.

4 · Muscles

Within the horse's body there are three different kinds of muscle. They vary in their construction because they serve three different functions. The greatest muscle mass, the flesh of the horse, as it were, is referred to as skeletal or striated muscle. It is responsible for the maintenance of posture, for movement and for breathing. Around 40 per cent of the horse's body-weight is skeletal muscle, with an even higher proportion in those breeds which have been evolved for speed. The second type of muscle is referred to as smooth muscle because, when examined under a microscope, it lacks the striped appearance of skeletal muscle. It is generally found in internal organs, such as along the gastrointestinal tract, the bladder and the uterus. It is also the type of muscle which forms the walls of the arteries. In all these situations, smooth muscle regulates the movement along the tube of the various contents of the organ concerned. Many colics, for instance, result from disturbances in the normal functioning of smooth muscle, and it is the abnormally excessive movements of the smooth muscle in the bowel wall which cause the pain associated with colic. The third type of muscle is that which makes up the walls of the heart. It has characteristics of both the other two types of muscle, with its main features due to its obvious need to be continually contracting and relaxing as it pumps blood through the body. In man it has been calculated that the heart contracts and relaxes about 2,500,000,000 times in a lifetime. In a horse living about 20 years, the number of pumping actions would be about 500,000,000 (about 50,000 times per day).

This chapter will consider the role of skeletal muscle in influencing locomotion. Its importance in both stride frequency and stride length, the end determinants of speed, can be seen in Table 3. These factors can be examined at either the gross or cellular level. For example, the natural frequency of the limbs can be ascertained by measuring muscle bulk. For some measurements it has been found that although the Thoroughbred does not have longer legs relative to its length than other horses, it has a greater mass of muscle around the hip joint which favours a higher natural frequency of its hindlimb in comparison with other horses. At the cellular level such a factor as the diameter of the individual fibres and their energy generating capacity are important.

Table 3   The importance of muscle in dictating running speed

Running speed

↑

Co-ordinated Gait

Stride Length	×	Stride Frequency
Leg Length		Natural Frequency of Limbs
Range of Movement of Joints		Mechanical Advantage of Muscles
Acceleration Capacity		Intrinsic Speed of Contractile Elements
Internal Muscle Structure		Repetivity of Limb Movements
		(dependent on energy supply)

The skeletal muscles of the body can produce a regulated force; it is not an all-or-nothing contraction. The mechanism which enables them to do this, and the ability to sustain such activity, are dependent on both the inherited, or genetic, properties of the muscle and on the adaptations which occur with the correct type of training.

How muscle is made up

If a muscle is taken out of the body and dissected, it can be seen that over 90 per cent of it is made up of muscle cells, which, because of their length, are referred to as fibres. The remaining 10 per cent comprises the nerves, the blood-vessels and the connective tissue which separates individual muscle fibres, etc (Fig 19). The connective tissue surrounding the muscle bundles merges into the tendons which attach the muscle to the bones. The bones act as the levers which translate the contraction of the muscles into movement of the horse's limbs and body. The blood-vessels which bring the blood into the muscles are, at first, relatively large. They then branch and branch again until they end up as small capillaries surrounding individual muscle cells and providing them with their fuel and oxygen. Blood does not flow through all these tiny vessels when the horse is at rest, but during strenuous exercise every last capillary will be utilised, with the result that blood flow may be increased by over sixty-fold. So that muscle cells can contract in an orderly pattern, each cell has a nerve coming to it. These nerves originate in the spinal cord, and they pass on to the muscle instructions coming from the brain to allow the co-ordinated action of the different muscle masses.

Unlike other cells in the horse's body, a muscle fibre has not one but many nuclei. These are spread out along its length, lying just beneath the outer covering (or membrane) of the fibre. This unusual structure is due to the fact that, during embryonic development, each muscle fibre

MUSCLE

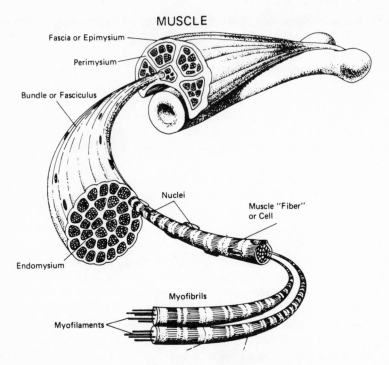

Fig 19 Basic structure of muscle. Epimysium, perimsium and endomysium are terms used to describe the connective (fibrous) tissue separating bundles of individual muscle fibres (From *Physiology of Exercise,* D.R. Lamb, Macmillan Publishing Co, New York, 1978)

develops from the fusion of 100-200 different immature muscle cells. The length and diameter of a muscle cell varies both within and between muscles. The actual size of the muscle itself is affected by both its normal growth and activity. When an increase in muscle mass occurs as a result of various activities, such as weight-lifting in man, this increase in size is brought about by the individual muscle fibres becoming larger (hypertrophy), rather than being due to the formation of any new cells (hyperplasia). As will become increasingly obvious, the indivual muscle fibre is extremely plastic, being able to alter according to its activity and its nutritional state. During periods of starvation muscle atrophies, or wastes away, as the protein within the fibres is broken down and taken to the liver. Here it is partially converted to glucose to provide fuels for the essential organs such as the brain.

To understand how each fibre can contract to create the power generated by a muscle, we have to look at how it is made up. As with all other cells, the major portion of the muscle cell is water (about 70 per cent).

Within this water lie the chemical substances necessary to produce contraction and the organelles (microscopic structures within the cell) which manufacture the substances which cause the contraction to occur in a regulated rather than a haphazard fashion. After water, the greatest part of the cell is taken up by the contractile machinery. This consists of hundreds of long rod-like structures which run parallel to the length of the fibre. Each rod-like structure is referred to as a myofibril, and is made up of about nine different proteins in a repeating pattern. Because of the way in which these repeating units of proteins, or sarcomeres, absorb light under the microscope, the myofibrils take on a cross-striated appearance (Plate 6), hence the name, striated muscle. When the muscle is at rest, each sarcomere within the myofibril is a constant length and so the length of the myofibril is dependent on the number of sarcomeres present. Growth of the muscle with age results in additional sarcomeres being added to the ends of the myofibrils.

Within the myofibrils are two kinds of even smaller filaments of differing thickness. They are arranged in such a way that they interdigitate with each other. They consist of two proteins: the one making up the thicker filaments is called myosin and the protein making up the thinner filaments is called actin. There are cross-bridges between the two types of filaments, and it is the changes in these cross-bridges which allow the thin actin fibres to slide between the myosin filaments and thus cause contraction of the muscle fibres.

In addition to the myofibrils within the muscle fibre, there are also other structures present which are necessary for the normal functions other than contraction. Under the membrane surrounding the fibres, and to a lesser extent between the myofibrils themselves, are the powerhouses of the cells, the mitochondria. These are the organelles within which the highly efficient aerobic combustion of fuels occurs, generating energy in the form of ATP. The number and size of these mitochondria can vary greatly between different fibres. There is also an organelle called the sarcoplasmic reticulum found throughout the muscle fibre. It is connected with the outer membrane of the fibre, and it runs between the myofibrils. Its purpose is to transmit quickly into the myofibrils the electrical signal which is triggered off by the arrival of a nerve impulse at the cell membrane. At the same time, calcium ions are released from vesicles, or storage chambers, within the sarcoplasmic reticulum.

Also dispersed throughout the fibres are fuel stores ready for energy production. As shown in Plate 7, there is an abundant supply of glycogen granules (the principal energy store) throughout the muscle cells. In association with these granules are the enzymes which partially break them down ready for the fuel to be used by the mitochondria. Small fat globules are also found around the mitrochondria, the exact numbers present varying greatly between individual fibres.

Although the precise mechanism of muscle contraction has still to be unfolded, much has already been discovered. The start of the process is the arrival of an impulse from a nerve. This creates an electrical signal at the membrane around the muscle fibre. The signal is quickly transmitted through the rest of the body of the fibre via the sarcoplasmic reticulum, which then releases calcium ions. These ions diffuse into the myofibrils and release the blocking action of a chemical which keeps the myofibrils relaxed. This in turn allows the myofilaments to be drawn between the myosin filaments by the action of the cross-bridges. The end result is a considerable shortening of the sarcomere, and an overall contraction of the muscle as a whole. As the actin becomes disconnected from the cross-bridges, relaxation occurs. The whole cycle of events requires energy in the form of ATP. When a high frequency of contractions is required, as in galloping, a very rapid turnover of ATP is also necessary.

When we look at the colour of muscles, it is obvious that they are not all the same. Some muscles are white and some are red. It is, however, even more complicated than you might think. Although the breast muscles of chickens are white, those of birds which migrate long distances are very red. Even within the same breed there can be differences. So, veal muscle is white, whereas in older animals allowed to move around freely it is red. These colour differences are due to the amounts of a protein called myoglobin which is present. Myoglobin is similar to haemoglobin, and it is responsible for carrying oxygen within the muscle cells. Cells rich in myoglobin are red, and those low in myoglobin are white. So the colour of a muscle is closely related to its capacity to use oxygen, ie its aerobic capacity. Naturally, muscles that are required for sustained activity (such as the breast muscles in migrating birds) are red, while those not adapted for activity at all (such as in veal calves) or for only short bursts of activity (as in the breast muscles of the chicken) are white.

Colour differences can be seen with the naked eye, but when a muscle is examined under a microscope, differences can be seen even in muscles which appear to be the same colour. This is because not all the fibres within the muscle have exactly the same make-up. They may have slightly different functions, or be used in different circumstances. Individual muscle cells can vary widely in their ability to use oxygen, and also in how frequently they can contract, ie some can contract more rapidly than others.

Muscle biopsy

In order to study the basic structure of the horse's muscles in situ, and to be able to determine the changes which may take place within a particular muscle as a result of training, racing, etc., a technique known as a muscle biopsy is used. This does not involve any pain for the animal, and causes it no lasting damage. In a 'percutaneous needle muscle biopsy' a 3-5mm diameter needle is inserted through a small incision in the skin. A local anaesthetic ensures that neither of these processes causes any pain. When the biopsy needle is withdrawn, it brings with it a piece of muscle weighing 100-200mg. This minute fragment is enough for numerous tests to be carried out on the properties and composition of the muscle. The technique is used extensively in man to study muscle disorders and in athletes. The small amount of muscle removed is replaced by new muscle fibres, not scar tissue, so there is no effect on the muscle's performance. When carrying out a biopsy, no more restraint is needed than when one is taking a blood sample. Over 1,500 biopsies in horses have been carried out by one of the authors without any untoward effects. The safety of the technique is further demonstrated by the fact that after biopsy, horses have even gone on to win Group 1 races. Many different muscles can be sampled using the biopsy needle, depending on what the study is concerned with. Most of the sampling in the horse is restricted to a muscle called the middle gluteal muscle, which lies over the hind quarters (Plate 8). This muscle is extremely large and is very important in generating the propulsive forces necessary for movement. It is thus a very convenient muscle to sample when looking at the effects of training, or possibly assessing the athletic potential of an animal.

Once this small piece of muscle has been obtained, it can be examined in different ways in order to look at the various aspects of muscle function. If the make-up of the different cells is to be studied, a technique known as histochemistry is used. This involves cutting very thin slices of muscle, about five-thousandths of a millimetre thick. These minute sections are then placed on a microscope slide for examination. The capacity to use oxygen, the amount of glycogen and fat present, and the relative speeds at which the fibres can contract, are all examples of information which can be obtained using various chemical stains to highlight specific features on such a slide. In other cases the muscle tissue is homogenised into a kind of 'soup' and the desired chemicals measured in the usual way. If we want to look at the very minute detail of the internal structure of muscle cells, samples are examined under an extremely powerful electron microscope which can magnify objects tens of thousands of times.

Identification of muscle fibre types

As has already been mentioned, the fibres within a muscle are not all identical. There are two common methods of differentiating fibres: those which distinguish them according to their relative contracting, or twitch, speeds and those which distinguish them by their ability to use oxygen, ie by their aerobic capacity. This latter measurement also identifies their capacity for sustained energy production. When looking at the twitch speeds, we use a stain which picks up an enzyme called myosin ATPase. This enzyme is responsible for the breakdown of ATP at the cross-bridges, and so large amounts present mean that a great deal of contraction is anticipated. The staining enables muscle fibres to be put into two groups: those which are slow contracting, the slow twitch fibres, and those which are fast contracting, the fast twitch fibres (Plate 9). The slow and fast twitch fibres are also referred to as Type I and Type II fibres. The Type II fibres can be further divided into Type IIA and IIB fibres, with the latter being able to contract slightly faster than the Type IIA fibres, but only being used when near maximal power outputs are required. The exact proportions of these differing types of fibres present are genetically determined, and to all intents and purposes they do not appear to be altered by training.

In most large mammals a mixture of these two fibre types are seen through the muscle. The proportions do, however, vary in different sites within the muscle and between different muscles which do different jobs. In general, the highest proportion of Type II fibres are found in the superficial, or outermost, parts of the muscle. In elite human athletes it has been shown that in the vastus lateralis (a key muscle of the thigh for running) a relationship exists between the proportion of these fibre types and prowess on the athletic track. Sprinters, for example, have a very high proportion of Type II fibres, whereas long-distance and marathon runners have a very high proportion of Type I fibres and can thus stand sustained activity without becoming fatigued. Middle-distance runners have approximately equal proportions of both types of fibre, as does the population as a whole. It would appear, then, that for outstanding success at sprinting or long-distance running, the correct genetic endowment is essential, with proper training developing this potential.

When the middle gluteal muscle of the horse is examined, it is found that, as in the vastus lateralis in man, a relationship exists between performance and the proportion of Type I and Type II fibres. The horse recently developed for sheer speed, the American racing quarterhorse, has almost entirely Type II fibres, whereas those horses which are able to sustain prolonged activity, such as those achieving success in endurance rides, have a higher proportion of Type I fibres (Table 4).

Table 4   Percentage of slow twitch fibres in different breeds

Quarterhorse	7
Thoroughbred	13
Arab	14
Standardbred	18
Shetland Pony	21
Pony	23
Donkey	24
Endurance horse, mostly of Arab breeding	28
Heavy Hunter	31

Further studies have been carried out to see if within a breed, such as the Thoroughbred, differences can be seen between sprinters and stayers. Although when groups of animals in both categories are compared there appears to be a statistical difference, a degree of overlap exists. This means that when an individual horse is sampled in order to assess its racing potential, some horses could be wrongly categorised if the evaluation was based solely on the proportion of Type I and Type II fibres. In addition, it goes without saying that numerous other physiological and psychological factors have a vital input.

As well as identifying fibres according to their contractile speed, they can also be differentiated by their metabolic properties, such as their ability to use oxygen or to break down glycogen. It is the fibres' varying ability to use oxygen which is measured when we look at the differences between fibres. For the sake of simplicity, fibres are considered to have either a high or a low oxidative ability (Plate 10). When we combine this factor with the contractile properties of muscle fibres, we find that we arrive at three distinct groups of fibres. These are the slow twitch, high-oxidative fibres (ST), the fast twitch, high-oxidative fibres (FTH) and the fast twitch, low-oxidative fibres (FT). The fact that all slow twitch fibres turn out to be highly oxidative is only to be expected from their function in the horse's body. They are in continual use maintaining posture and controlling body activity. Similarly, the oxidative differences between the two types of fast twitch or Type II fibres also reflect differences in function.

The oxidative ability of a muscle fibre can be altered by training. When a horse is being trained, the oxidative capacity increases, whereas during long periods of inactivity it decreases. So, increasing oxidative capacity is one of the effects aimed for in training, as will be discussed later. The higher a fibre's oxidative capacity, the greater the ability of the fibre to generate ATP aerobically rather than anaerobically (which can quickly tire the fibre). In parallel with any changes in the oxidative capacity of a fibre, there are also changes in the number of small blood-vessels, or capillaries, around each fibre. Those fibres with the highest oxidative capacity have the most abundant capillary supply, so that the amount of oxygen supplied by the blood can match the potential of the fibres to use it. The characteristics of the different fibre types are summarised in Table 5.

Table 5   Characteristics of muscle fibre types in the horse

	Type 1 (slow)	Type II (fast)	
	ST	FTH	FT
Speed of contraction	Slow	Fast	Fast
Maximum tension developed	Low	High	High
Myosin ATPase activity	Low	High	High
Oxidative capacity	High	Intermediate to High	Low
Number of capillaries	High	Intermediate	Low
Enzymes for glucose breakdown	Intermediate	High	High
Enzymes for free fatty acid breakdown	High	Intermediate	Low
Fatiguability	Low	Intermediate	High

So far, we have seen that the contractile characteristics of a muscle are important in determining performance potential, and the oxidative capacity is important in helping the horse to achieve this potential. In sprinters, the size of the muscle and the diameter of the individual fibres are also important. This is because the amount of power output that can be obtained from a muscle is dependent on the muscle's size. If we compare a Quarterhorse with a Standardbred, for example, the former has much bulkier muscles than the latter, just as the human sprinter is more muscular than a marathon runner. This greater muscle bulk is due to both a greater number of fibres within the muscle and also to the fact that each fibre has a greater diameter. Both factors are probably genetically determined, although the fibre diameter can be influenced by correct training methods such as weight-lifting in human athletes. If, however, the muscle fibres are large in order to produce high power outputs, they have a low oxidative capacity because most of the fibre is occupied with myofibrils rather than mitochondria. This is the reason why fatigue occurs rapidly in sprinters, who can only maintain high power outputs for very short periods.

Recruitment of muscle fibres
Now that the different types of muscle fibre have been described, their significance can be considered in further detail. During most muscle contractions it is unnecessary for the muscle to generate maximum power, and so not all the fibres need to be stimulated. An orderly, rather than haphazard, selection of fibres is, however, necessary. This selection

is regulated by the pattern of nerve impulses reaching the muscle fibres from the spinal cord. To maintain posture or to walk, only the nerves supplying slow twitch, and possibly some fast twitch, high oxidative, fibres will be used. This is because only about 10 per cent of the fibres will need to contract in order to produce the necessary power. As the horse increases its speed, and more and more power is required, an increasing proportion of fibres contract as more and more nerves are stimulated. So, at a medium trot, approximately 50 per cent of fibres are contracting, involving all the slow twitch and many of the fast twitch, high-oxidative fibres. At the full gallop all the fibres have to contract, as shown in Plate 11.

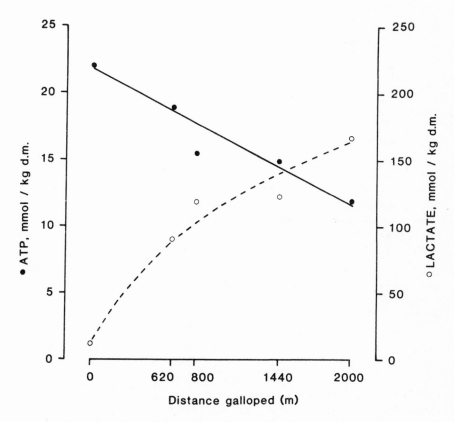

Fig 20 The extent of decrease in ATP and increase in lactate in muscle with increasing distance at maximal speeds

Causes of fatigue

As we all know, our ability to continue at a required level of performance is limited by the onset of fatigue. For mental activities, it appears that the origin of fatigue lies in the brain, and muscle fatigue starts largely within the muscle involved. When trying to determine the causes of fatigue and how best to delay its onset, we must consider the type of exercise involved because the fatigue resulting from maximal effort is different from that experienced by horses involved in endurance rides. It should be appreciated that fatigue is an early warning sign to the body that it has to slow down. It is a protective device to prevent the more severe state of exhaustion where medical treatment becomes necessary.

The causes of fatigue during exercise can be summarised as follows:

1 The accumulation of lactic acid within fibres during maximal exercise.
2 The using up of muscle glycogen stores during prolonged submaximal exercise.
3 Dehydration due to excessive sweating, leading in turn to a drop in blood volume and poor blood flow to muscles and other organs.
4 Lameness, altering the normal gait and placing abnormal strains on muscle and bones.

During short-term maximal exercise, where all, or nearly all, the muscle fibres are recruited, fatigue results from an accumulation of lactic acid in some of the fibres. These fibres are then unable to maintain normal contractions. The fibres which are most prone to the build-up of lactic acid are those that are only recruited at the faster speeds, as they also have the lowest oxidative capacity. What happens is that as these fibres are utilised, the high turnover of ATP which they need cannot be met by aerobic means, and so (as was discussed earlier) the ATP supplies have to be replenished by anaerobic metabolism as well. As the phosphocreatine which is involved in this is rapidly used up, lactic acid has to be produced to help maintain ATP requirements. The lactic acid is formed so rapidly that it cannot pass into the bloodstream quickly enough, and so there is a build-up of the acid in the fibres. Because it is an acid, there is an increase in acidity (which may also also be referred to as a drop in pH) in the cell. A point is reached when the muscle fibre can no longer function properly and ceases normal contractions. When this occurs, the number of fibres available to contract decreases, and so both the power output and the speed of movement decrease. The fall off in speed depends on the proportion of muscle fibres affected. It is this build-up of lactate within muscles that is probably responsible for the 'fading' of many horses during the last furlong (200m) of a race.

The production of lactate may also cause pain in its own right, so the horse's ability to continue performing may depend, to some extent, on its response to pain and its willingness to carry on performing in the face of pain. This may be an important factor when the winning post is near, and may make all the difference between struggling on to win and just accepting defeat. The speed at which fatigue occurs is dependent on the fitness of the horse. The fitter the horse, the greater the aerobic capacity of its muscle fibres and the less reliance it will have to place on lactate production to produce the large amounts of ATP needed. In an unfit horse a higher proportion of low oxidative fibres will be present, so lactic-acid accumulation will occur at lower speeds as these fibres have to be brought into action. Once the accumulated lactate has been removed from the muscle fibre (a process which may take over an hour), exercise can then be continued at the original fast pace. The removal of lactate can be more readily achieved if the horse continues to perform mild exercise after the gallop, rather than being completely rested. Whether the more rapid removal of the lactate is actually beneficial, other than enabling the horse to perform again sooner that same day, is not yet known.

Recent studies at Newmarket have shown that during this high build-up of lactic acid in the horse's muscle there is a marked decrease in the amount of ATP in the muscle. This was surprising because previously most work had indicated that supplies of ATP were maintained despite a build-up of lactic acid. These older studies were carried out in man and laboratory animals, and it appears that the horse can accumulate more lactic acid than these species. The decrease in ATP appears to be related to the actual amount of lactic acid which accumulates. As shown in Fig 20, the further the horse runs at maximum speed, the less ATP there is. At the same time the quantity of the other phosphagen, creatine phosphate, is also very low. Human exercise physiology books report that these phosphagen stores are restored within minutes. In the horse, however, it may take an hour for them to return to normal values after strenuous exercise. So, we can conclude that, although horses are able to have a higher anaerobic energy production than man, their recovery period afterwards is longer. This also applies to the time taken to remove lactate after exercise.

As prolonged exercise is usually performed at speeds which are well below maximal levels, anaerobic metabolism is not necessary for the production of sufficient ATP in these circumstances. The accumulation of lactic acid is not, therefore, a problem either. Instead, a mixture of fuels, ie approximately equal amounts of glycogen and free fatty acids, is used at such aerobic workloads. The cause of fatigue in this situation is the consumption of all the glycogen stored within the muscle fibres and within the liver. When this happens insufficient fuel is available to generate the ATP requirements at all but the lowest speeds. Earlier, it was mentioned that at a trot, the pace of most endurance rides, only about half of the muscle fibres have to contract to produce sufficient power for movement. One might, therefore, expect a muscle biopsy taken at the end of such a ride to show an appreciable amount of glycogen still available. This is not the case. Biopsies show that all the fibres have lost the vast majority of their glycogen (Plate 10). This occurs because when the fibres normally used at this level of exercise consume all their glycogen, other fibres are brought into work. The slow twitch and fast twitch, high-oxidative fibres run out of glycogen first, followed eventually by the fast twitch, low oxidative fibres. When all of these are depleted, the horse still does not have to come to a complete standstill. A slower pace can still be maintained because some fuel can be supplied to the muscle cells in the form of free fatty acids from the blood circulation. The rate at which these free fatty acids can reach the muscle is insufficient to provide the energy for high speeds, but there are sufficient fat stores within the body for the horse to keep on at this slow pace for several days.

This inability to maintain their initial constant speed is often experienced by marathon runners at about 20 miles (32km) into the race, and they find that they, too, have to slow down. It has been referred to as 'hitting the wall'. At this point the human athlete feels pain as a warning sign to slow down. Whether horses experience the same sensations is unknown, but it is quite possible that those horses with 'heart' may try to ignore these signs and therefore cause severe damage to their muscles. It is the job of the astute rider to be able to detect any small sign that may indicate fatigue, and then to slow the horse down rather than have such decreased performance forced upon him later. As is well known, muscle fatigue is one of the most common causes of lameness in joints and muscles because co-ordination of movement is lost in fatigue, resulting in a careless and possibly disastrous movement. One practical way of detecting fatigue is to monitor heart rates during exercise using one of the heart-rate monitors commercially available and described in another chapter. Any increases in heart rate when going at a constant pace indicate that more effort is being required and that all is not well.

As glycogen depletion is the cause of fatigue in this type of exercise, several strategies can be used to increase the duration of exercise before fatigue occurs. First, a higher proportion of free fatty acids can be burnt. This may be brought about by either reducing speed, which is obviously undesirable in competitions, or by increasing the proportion utilised at the desired speed. As will be discussed shortly, this can be achieved through increasing fitness, and results in what is referred to as a glycogen sparing effect. The second important mechanism which can be used is the obvious one of increasing the amount of glycogen within the muscle cells. This strategy is used in marathon runners when they have their 'pasta parties' prior to a competition. They consume large quantities of carbohydrate, building up muscle supplies. However, in doing this it has to be realised that for every gram of glycogen stored up in the muscle, 3g of water will also be stored. So some athletes find that large amounts of glycogen stored within their muscle cells make their legs uncomfortable and heavy to lift. Whether extra glycogen stores can be added to a horse's muscle as a result of diet changes has only been studied to a limited extent, and the results are far from definite one way or the other. However, as the horse has naturally high levels of muscle glycogen (about 50 per cent more than in man), it is unlikely that any additional glycogen can be added to the muscles of a horse which has been on a correct high-energy diet. Even if it was possible, it may not necessarily be desirable.

In contrast to recovery from maximal exercise, recovery from fatigue following prolonged submaximal exercise is a much slower process. As illustrated in Plate 12, it takes up to several days for the glycogen stores to be completely restored to normal. Whether high carbohydrate diets can result in a faster recovery is still the subject of research. Preliminary results indicate the importance of ensuring adequate carbohydrate supplies to at least hasten the early stages of replacement. This is an important consideration in an endurance ride lasting over several days. As discussed elsewhere, as well as replenishing glycogen supplies it is also important to replace fluid and electrolytes lost during such endurance competitions.

While on the subject of glycogen, over the past few years there has developed a belief among some racehorse trainers that glycogen stores may be the limiting factor during short races of 1-2 miles (1,600-3,200m). From all the evidence available this is not the case, as only about half the glycogen is utilised during such races, and most of that is used during the initial stages of the race. Once again, then, it appears that as long as the horse is on a normal high-energy ration there appears to be no necessity to try to use glycogen loading techniques.

Adaptations with training

Increasing fitness can only be obtained as a result of training of one sort or another. The fitness needed for a competition will vary greatly. For instance, the fitness required for a novice one-day event is not as great as that for a top-class three-day event. Whatever the competition the horse is aimed at, its fitness should allow the horse to complete the competition in the desired manner without the development of fatigue. Fitness involves the tuning up of all the body systems so that they can give a well-regulated response to the task they face. It is pointless to get some of the body systems fit and others not, as breakdown will occur at the weakest point.

Of the body's systems, probably most is known about how the muscles adapt during training and inactivity. With training, the extent of the alterations within the muscles are largely dependent on the pattern and frequency of the nerve impulses arriving at the individual muscle fibres. Therefore, one can only get a favourable effect from training if it entails the same type and intensity of exercise as that which will be encountered during competition. For instance, the fast twitch, low-oxidative fibres are only recruited during high intensity exercise, and if speed is required during the competition, then sufficient sprinting should be included in the training programme. If the competition requires exercise below or just above the anaerobic threshold, then prolonged exercise at these levels will be needed to increase the oxidative capacity of the muscles. This increased oxidative capacity is needed both to increase the amount of exercise that can be undertaken before the onset of fatigue, and also to raise the speed at which anaerobic metabolism becomes important.

The adaptation of muscle with training can be studied by looking at muscle under a microscope or in a test tube. Although under artificial experimental conditions it is possible to alter the proportions of Type I (slow) and Type II (fast) fibres present, this does not occur under normal training conditions. Within the Type II fibres, however, it can be shown that a changeover occurs from Type IIB to Type IIA and vice versa, depending on the training being undertaken. The most marked alterations within the muscle fibres during training are those related to their metabolic properties. Training always results in an increase in the fibre's ability to utilise oxygen, ie more and larger mitochondria are built that contain more of the enzymes responsible for the combustion of glycogen and free fatty acids (see Plate 13). With a lot of high-intensity training, all the fibres develop a high-aerobic capacity. The same effect can also be achieved, however, with prolonged training at intermediate speeds, because the fibres which are initially involved at the slower speeds eventually use up all their glycogen, and the rest of the fibres then have to be recruited into action. In conjunction with this increase in the levels of enzymes within the mitochondria, there is also an increase in the level of enzymes responsible for supplying and degrading free fatty acids before they enter the mitochondria. This results in the favourable effect referred to earlier, namely, that more free fatty acids can now be utilised. As most research indicates that little change occurs in the enzymes responsible for the breakdown of glycogen or glucose, there is a proportionally greater utilisation of free fatty acids at any given workload. This is the glycogen sparing effect so important in improving performance.

In line with this increase in the capacity to utilise oxygen, there is also an increase in the number of small capillaries around the muscle fibres so that the increased oxidative potential of the fibres can be properly utilised. During periods of inactivity, a reversal of the increased oxidative capacity occurs, leading to a reduced ability to perform exercise and a return to unfitness. Interestingly, the little evidence that is available suggests that the effects of inactivity are slower to become apparent in horses than they are in man. So, box rest of even several weeks is unlikely to cause much change in the fitness of a horse. It also would appear that this aerobic fitness may be better maintained in older horses than in young ones.

As has already been mentioned, when the energy requirements for exercise cannot be met by aerobic metabolism, extra energy is produced by the formation of lactic acid. As will be appreciated from what has already been written, the exact timing of this change in the source of energy production will vary between different horses depending on the oxidative capacity of their muscles. This point has been called the anaerobic threshold, or the point of Onset of Blood Lactate Accumulation (OBLA). These terms are used to indicate the work intensity at which there is a sudden increase in the concentration of lactate in the blood. The work intensity at which this occurs is considerably increased after training (see Chapter 8). When the capacity of human athletes has been assessed for endurance events, a high correlation has been found between the anaerobic threshold and performance.

In the human athlete such research is carried out by the athlete running on a treadmill, or by working on a bicycle ergometer at four or five different workloads of increasing intensity. Each workload is performed for several minutes before a blood sample is taken and the next workload commenced. From the results a plot is obtained and the point of anaerobic threshold is calculated. A few similar studies have been carried out in horses on a high-speed treadmill. Other tests, using trotters working at different speeds on the track, also indicated that the horses with the higher anaerobic threshold were the ones considered by their trainer to be the better performers.

Perhaps now is the time to issue a cautionary warning to those who, having read some of the less informed articles about interval training and about the necessity for more and more work, want to put such schemes into use. Although it is often highly desirable to cause a marked increase in oxidative capacity, this is not always the case. As stated earlier, it is important to train for the particular competition in mind. Although it has been shown that increased aerobic capacity, and hence a higher anaerobic threshold, is desirable for endurance athletes so that they can maintain higher speeds, this is not the case for athletes competing in events lasting only several minutes, and especially not in sprinting events where a higher power output is required. For assessing fitness and potential for these events, other tests which measure actual power output have been developed. The reason for this difference in requirements is that when fibres become more highly aerobic, rather than becoming larger, as occurs with strength training, there appears to be an actual decrease in fibre diameter of those cells which were originally low-oxidative fibres. The result is that all fibres, no matter what their type, end up with a similar diameter. This decrease in size of some fibres is to allow a better diffusion of oxygen throughout the fibre so that the now enlarged mitochrondria can be adequately oxygenated. So, as you improve the horse's anaerobic threshold, you lose power because power is directly proportional to the diameter of the muscle fibres involved. You cannot train for both extreme endurance and pure speed. This explains why horses may have a key distance over which they perform most successfully, and also why true stayers cannot be sprinters and vice versa. Training methods have to be tailored to the individual. Too much emphasis on interval training at high speeds will increase stamina but reduce strength and ability to accelerate rapidly.

Tying-up, set-fast, azoturia
Fortunately, actual muscle disease in the horse is rare. The exception is a condition brought on by exercise which has the scientific name of exertional rhabdomyolysis. This is better known as tying-up, azoturia, set-fast or Monday morning disease. All these terms describe variations in the clinical picture of the same basic condition. For example, tying-up is often described as a milder form of azoturia. Exertional rhab-

Plate 6 High power photomicrograph of part of a muscle fibre showing the striations on the myofibrils, the proteins responsible for the contraction of the fibre. M = mitochondrion. From Exercise and Training D. H. Snow in Horse Management Ed. J. Hickman Academic Press, London 1984

Plate 7 High power photomicrograph showing the fuels within the muscle fibre. G = glycogen granules, L = lipid (fat) droplets, M = mitochondrion. From Exercise and Training D. H. Snow in Horse Management Ed. J. Hickman Academic Press, London 1984

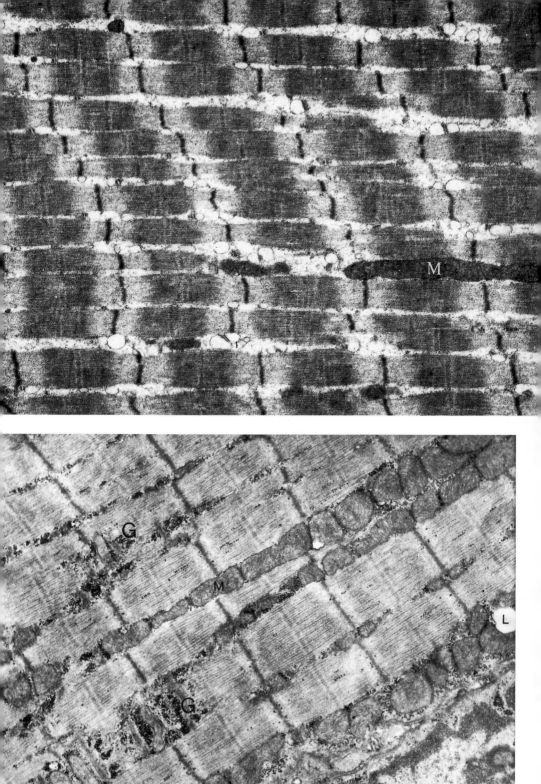

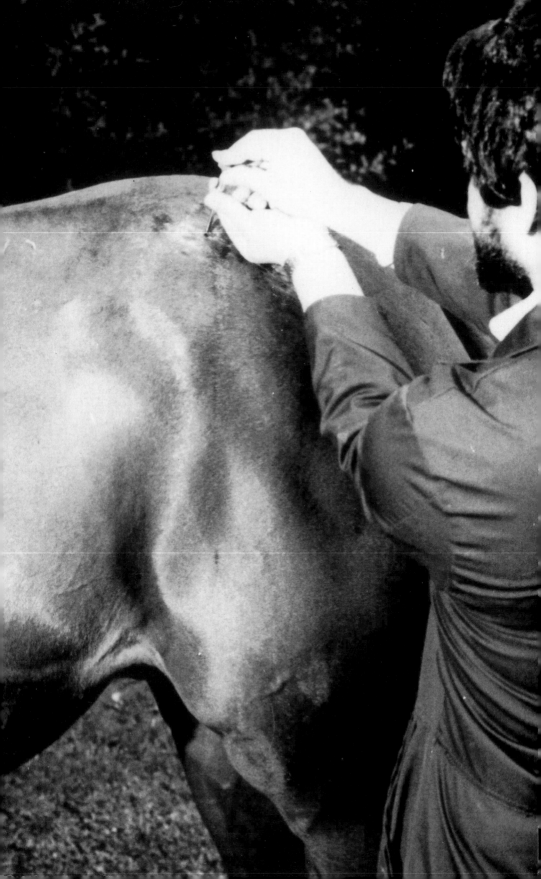

domyolysis is really a syndrome rather than a precise condition, and probably has a number of different triggering factors.

The condition is almost always brought on by exercise, either during or immediately afterwards. Its severity can vary from a slight stiffness or shortening of stride, to total inability to move and even recumbency. The muscles affected are usually those of the croup, loin and thigh of both sides of the body. Very occasionally the muscles of the foreleg, or of just one side of the body, may be involved. Pressure on the muscles shows them to be firm, swollen and painful. In severe cases, such pressure causes obvious distress to the animal resulting in a rise in its pulse rate, respiratory rate and temperature. Varying degrees of sweating and colic are seen in horses suffering from the condition, and they often have difficulty in passing urine. When they succeed in doing so, the urine may be discoloured owing to myoglobin from the broken down muscle cells being excreted via the kidneys.

The syndrome occurs in all breeds, ages and sexes. Having said that, in racing stables there appears to be a higher incidence in young fillies which may be related to hormonal and temperamental differences between fillies and colts or geldings. The cause of the condition is still largely unknown. In the 1930s it was suggested that very high levels of glycogen within the muscles triggered the condition because it was often seen on Mondays in Draught Horses after they had been rested on Sunday, but still given a high-grain diet. Although high-energy diets given to horses not in work undoubtedly do help precipitate the condition, they are not the entire story. Nevertheless, a horse's grain intake should always be reduced on days of inactivity, especially when the horse is only ridden out occasionally. As well as reducing the energy content of the diet in horses that continually suffer from attacks of tying-up, long slow warm-up periods are often also useful.

Investigations at the Animal Health Trust in Newmarket indicate that electrolyte imbalances may also predispose horses to attacks of exertional rhabdomyolysis. These may be imbalances of either sodium and potassium or of calcium and phosphate. Diagnosis of such cases requires the collection of simultaneous blood and urine samples. Once any imbalances have been corrected the problem is often cured.

Proper assessment, treatment and prevention of the condition depends on advice from your veterinary surgeon. Immediate treatment will largely depend on the severity of the condition, but is basically aimed at alleviating the causes of distress. Stopping all exercise prevents any further muscle damage. Assessing the severity of the condi-

Plate 8 Taking a muscle biopsy from the middle gluteal

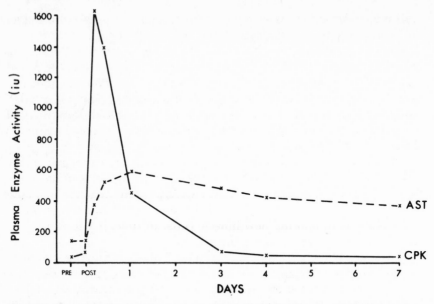

Fig 21 Pattern of changes in plasma enzyme activities following an attack of tying up

tion, and how it is responding to treatment, depends on the measurement of two or three enzymes in blood samples taken from the horse. These enzymes are creatine phosphokinase (CPK), aspartate aminotransferase (AST), and lactate dehydrogenase (LDH). After a single severe attack of the disease, the levels of CPK will peak within six to twelve hours (possibly increasing a hundred-fold), and then rapidly return to normal. AST takes longer to peak, and can take several weeks to return to normal. (Fig 21). The horse should not be given any exercise until the muscle enzymes have returned to normal, otherwise there is a danger of causing further muscle damage. If damage to the muscle is still occurring, the CPK level will remain elevated for a much longer period. It is also worth pointing out that CPK levels can also rise in an unfit animal after a hard bout of exercise, without any clinical evidence of tying-up. As has been pointed out elsewhere, measurement of CPK may be a useful aid in assessment of fitness.

Torn muscles and their treatment
One of the commonest injuries of the athletic horse is a 'torn muscle'. This phrase probably covers a whole group of problems. In some cases, the belly of the muscle will have been over-stretched, with the result that the individual muscle fibres are torn apart. When this happens, the

cell membranes of some of the cells will be damaged, and some of the cellular contents will leak out into the muscular tissue. The horse's body then recognises that it has a problem, and the normal inflammatory response gets under way. From the superficial point of view, this means that a torn muscle shows the classical signs of inflammation; it is hot, swollen and painful. At the microscopic level, there is increased tissue fluid, perhaps mixed with blood if some of the small blood-vessels have also been ruptured. There are macrophages, the cellular equivalent of refuse collectors because they engulf and destroy damaged tissue. Within a relatively short time there will also be the early elements of muscle tissue repair. These will include collagen fibres, which make up a high proportion of scar tissue in an attempt to stabilise the weakened area. The horse is, therefore, far more interested in stabilising the muscle than it is in making new muscle cells. In time, it will replace the damaged muscle cells. Of all the tissues of the body, muscle replaces itself more readily than any other except the skin. The problem for the athlete is that by the time all the new muscle cells have been formed, etc, the repair process will have become almost a fixture. Bundles of collagen fibres forming adhesions to surrounding muscle fibres (and so limiting their movement) do not help normal muscle function.

The clinical condition recognised as a torn muscle may not be limited to the muscle itself. In many cases it will also involve, to a greater or lesser extent, the tendon by which the muscle is attached to the bony lever which it has to move. Because tendons have such high tensile strength, the point where the tendon and the muscle join together is often more likely to be damaged during over-stretching than the tendon itself. The result is that a strained muscle may involve tearing of the fibrous sheath around the muscle, release of large amounts of blood into the area from blood-vessels damaged where they lead into the area, and general weakening of the junction between muscle and tendon. The difficulty is how to solve the problem in order to enable normal athletic function to be regained as quickly as possible.

Even from the earliest times it was realised that rubbing such injuries made the horse feel better. As we can tell when we rub one of our own muscles, it increases the superficial blood supply to the area (as shown by the skin becoming redder), and so presumably this increased blood supply can result in a more rapid mobilisation of the body's healing process. In addition, the increased blood supply makes the area feel warmer, and this appears to reduce the amount of pain felt. 'Strapping' a horse, which consists of slapping the muscles with a leather strap, or rubbing the horse vigorously with straw, was one of the early forms of preventive medicine. The groom strapped the horse after violent exercise, such as a hard day's hunting, in order to speed up the healing of any bruising and tearing which had taken place in the large muscle masses of the body. Mechanical means can also be used to induce the same effect. Niagara therapy is the use of a three-dimensional circular movement of the machine to speed up the removal of the leaked fluids, etc from the area by increasing the local blood circulation. The vibrations produced are perfectly safe, even in unskilled hands. They also seem to penetrate effectively through the horse's body. So, if you apply a unit to one side of a horse's upper leg, you can feel the vibrations with your other hand on the other side of the leg. Like strapping and good grooming, the larger Niagara units might have a role to play in stimulating the blood supply to 'cold' muscles before a competition.

Another form of physiotherapy which is sometimes used in the treatment of torn muscles is faradism. This consists of applying a localised electrical current to a muscle in order to produce the same effect on the muscle fibres as the electrical impulse which is produced at the nerve endings. Each time the current is passed, the muscles in the area contract. The contractions set up a pumping effect to drain fluids, etc away from the area (Plate 14). Faradism only stimulates muscles, and is not used on other kinds of injury. The current is applied by fixing a large electrode in continuous contact with the skin (often by means of a 'roller' around the horse's chest) and then applying another, small, electrode to the affected area. Fluids, such as water or saline, or special gels are used to ensure a good electrical contact between the electrode and the horse's skin. When you stimulate an injured muscle and make it contract, it hurts the horse. Careful observation on the part of the operator will therefore enable the affected area to be ascertained. So, faradism has a diagnostic role. It should never be the only diagnostic method used on an injury, however, because it does only relate to pain felt when a muscle contracts. A broken bone will cause pain when a muscle attached to it contracts, but faradism cannot diagnose whether it is an injured muscle or a broken bone which we are dealing with. When faradism is used in the treatment of muscle injuries, the aim is to get the muscles contracting gently and rhythmically. If too strong a current is used, faradism is very painful. Instead of helping healing it can then cause further tearing and damage. It follows that this technique is best left entirely in skilled hands. When applied to a damaged muscle for up to thirty minutes per day, faradism used properly can prevent the development of new adhesions in the muscle and gradually break down the adhesions which have already formed.

Whereas faradism is restricted to the treatment of muscular injuries, ultrasound has a far more general application. It is a technique which is widely used by physiotherapists in both the human and equine fields to treat trauma to soft tissues and bone, joint problems, localised circulatory disorders, etc. The name is derived from the fact that it utilises sound waves which are above the 17,000 cycles per second which the human ear can detect. In fact, the range used therapeutically is usually between 500,000 and 3 million cycles per second. The sound waves are produced by using a high-frequency current to cause mechanical vibrations within the machine, but unlike Niagara therapy where it is the vibrations which are used, in this case it is the sound produced during the vibration which is utilised. To be really effective, ultrasound requires the ultrasound head to be applied to skin which has been shaved and coated with a gel to ensure air-free contact with the skin. In the horse shaving is usually omitted, so some loss of efficiency is inevitable. Treatment is usually carried out for three to ten minutes daily.

Ultrasound has been said to work in a number of ways. As the sound waves pass through a medium such as muscle tissue, they stimulate energy release. Certainly, ultrasound can produce a temperature rise in the treated area. In man this can result in tissue temperatures of 104-113°F (40-45°C). It is thought that this heat can result in increased blood flow and some degree of analgesia, or pain relief. It also tends to relax muscle tension. Ultrasound treatment of tendons is said to decrease their spasticity and allow them to be more elastic in function. In all tissues the sound energy may increase the rate of tissue repair by increasing the rate of protein synthesis. Although the technique is widely used, there is a lack of conclusive evidence that it does work. In a paper to a British Equine Veterinary Association meeting, Bradley claimed that tests carried out in a large human hospital showed that the results obtained with ultrasound were as good or better if the machine was not switched on during the therapy!

At the present time there is an increasing amount of interest in the use of low-power cold lasers to treat soft-tissue injuries to muscles, etc. The laser is usually a gallium-aluminium-arsenide semiconductor laser which emits light in the infra-red spectrum. The light is pulsed, with up to 360 pulses per second (Plate 15). In some machines the light is emitted as a very narrow beam so that several crystals have to be grouped together to give a spread of light over an appreciable area. There is, however, one machine which has solved this problem optically, and which emits a 2 × 1in (50 × 25mm) beam. These lasers are perfectly safe, as long as they are not shone directly into the eyes. They do not burn holes into the horses (or the operators!) and indeed you cannot see or feel anything being emitted at all. Thankfully, the machines include an infra-red test cell so that one can make sure that everything is actually working. The clinical evidence which is accumulating about their use indicates that while such lasers are not a panacea for all soft-tissue injuries, they are a very valuable form of therapy. One word of warning: laser treatment will often produce a cosmetic cure, ie the muscle or tendon will look completely normal. It does not follow however, that the internal structures are completely returned to their normal state. A period of rest will still be necessary in many cases, even if the rest can be much shorter than would otherwise be the case.

New treatments, especially invisible new treatments, should always be taken with a pinch of salt unless one can prove how they work. The effect of a cold laser on some of the hormones which are responsible for the classic symptoms of inflammation has been investigated at the New Bolton Center in the USA. The effect of a working laser and a placebo which did not emit anything were examined in relation to cortisol (the natural corticosteroid which is released as a response to stress), adrenocorticotropic hormone (released during inflammatory conditions), and serotonin (which constricts the swollen blood-vessels in inflamed areas and so also reduces pain). Their results showed a statistically significant increase in the levels of serotonin circulating four hours after laser treatment compared with the placebo. Cortisol levels were significantly reduced. It appears, therefore, that laser therapy does have a measurable effect to reduce inflammation via the controlling hormones associated with it. Despite this, it remains to be seen whether a potentially valuable form of therapy will fall into disrepute because of the ease with which it can be carried out by untrained lay operators who are unable first to make an accurate diagnosis of what they are actually treating.

5 · The Horse's Life Blood: How its Internal Transport System Works

The cardiovascular system is the body's transport system. The blood-vessels are the routes along which various chemical substances can be transported either dissolved in the blood or linked to the blood cells. The cells themselves can also be transported to areas where they are most needed. There are two main types of blood-vessel: arteries and veins. As a general rule, the arteries bring the blood to the various parts of the body and the veins take the blood back to start its journey all over again. When the blood passes along the arteries, it is being pushed along under pressure. Indeed, there are some muscles in the arterial walls which help maintain the pumping action. When the blood passes along the veins, it is draining passively and is only at a low pressure. So, if a horse cuts an artery, the blood will spurt out rhythmically for quite a distance but if a vein is cut the blood merely drains out in a steady stream. Where the arteries end and the veins start there are very fine blood-vessels called capillaries. Not all the capillaries in a given part of the horse's body will be in use at any one time. When there is reduced demand for blood and all that it brings with it, a proportion of the capillaries will be shut down. At exercise, however, when the horse needs all the oxygen, fuels, etc, that it can get, then the whole capillary bed to the muscles will be opened up and utilised.

The transport system is powered by the heart. Although the structure of the horse's heart is basically no different from that of any other mammal, it may be considered to have a direct effect on the horse's monetary value because the horse is kept, in many cases, for performance rather than meat. So a heart defect in a cow is less likely to affect the reason why we keep that cow than will a heart defect in a horse. There will, of course, be many occasions when a horse's performance is limited by the ability of its heart to function. This does not necessarily mean that the horse's performance is curtailed by any pathological fault in the heart, merely that one horse's heart may not achieve the same output as its competitors'.

The heart is a double pump which has two major variables in its performance. First, the size of the pump can vary, and secondly the rate of pumping can vary. As we will show later, variations in the size of the pump only occur slowly. Variations in the rate of pumping, on the other hand, can occur rapidly.

The heart provides the pumping force for two parallel systems: the blood flow through the lungs and the blood flow to the rest of the body. These two systems interlock, rather like two interlocking rings (Fig 22). The left and right sides of the heart do completely separate jobs, but they have to be accurately synchronised. The left side of the heart pumps the blood out around the general circulation. As has been mentioned, the blood is first distributed to the various regions of the body in the arteries. These are continuously dividing into smaller and smaller arteries until they reach the capillary bed. It is the capillaries which are responsible for the blood being in intimate contact with the tissues which need its nourishment. The blood then flows back towards the heart in the veins, eventually entering the right side of the heart. From here it is pumped through the lungs before returning via the pulmonary

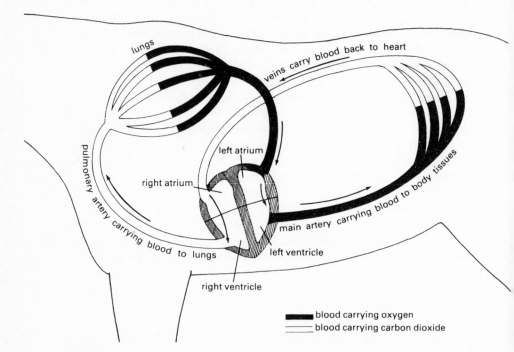

Fig 22 Schematic diagram illustrating the dual circulatory system, one part taking oxygenated blood to the tissue (systemic system), the other blood to the lungs for reoxygenation (pulmonary system)

veins to the left side of the heart again. Within the lungs the blood takes up oxygen and disposes of carbon dioxide, the main waste product of tissue metabolism. It is a very clever arrangement because it provides two distinct circulations but they both use the same blood. Each side of the heart has various sets of valves in order to divide the pump into two parts called the atrium and the ventricle. Between the right atrium and the right ventricle there is the tricuspid valve, so called because it has three cusps or flaps. When this is closed it prevents blood escaping backwards out of the right ventricle during ventricular contraction. All the blood is then pushed out of the ventricle through the pulmonary valve. On the left side of the heart, the atrium and ventricle are separated by the bicuspid valve, while the exit from the left ventricle is guarded by the aortic valve.

The actual pumping is achieved by co-ordinating the opening and closing of the valves with the contraction of the muscles around each chamber of the heart. The left ventricle, for example, fills up with blood when both the bicuspid valve is open and the wall of the left atrium contracts to expel the blood. The bicuspid valve then has to close before the ventricle empties, otherwise some of the blood would be pushed backwards into the atrium again. This is exactly what happens with certain physical abnormalities of the heart valves which prevent the valves from closing properly. If such leakage of blood back along the system occurs with the left side of the heart, it results in there being more blood held up in the circulation around the lungs than there should be, and this blood is at a higher than normal pressure. The end result is often to allow tissue fluid to escape out of the stretched walls of the blood-vessels into the surrounding tissues. This produces pulmonary oedema, and severely reduces the horse's athletic capabilities. Assuming, however, that the bicuspid valve closes normally, the contraction of the ventricular muscles and the opening of the aortic valve will push the blood out into the general circulation. The muscles of the left side of the heart are much better developed than those of the right side. This is because they have to pump the blood around the general circulation, and the pressure needed to do so is much greater than that needed to pump blood just around the lungs.

Heart sounds and murmurs

The use of a stethoscope enables you to hear the sounds made when the various valves of the pumping system open and close. The sounds are usually likened to 'lub dub', ie you are listening to two heart sounds. There are actually four heart sounds, and the slower the resting heart beat is, the more likely you are to hear all four of them. To understand exactly what you are listening to, it is necessary to know what is going on inside the heart during pumping. The first sound (the 'lub' sound) is associated with the closure of the tricuspid and bicuspid valves between the atria and the ventricles. The second sound (the 'dub' sound) is associated with the closure of the pulmonary and aortic valves. We mentioned earlier that there were, in fact, four heart sounds. The third heart sound follows immediately after the second sound and is associated with the filling of the ventricles with blood. The fourth heart sound actually comes immediately before the first sound, and is associated with the contraction of the walls of the two atria. The gap between the first and second heart sounds is called systole, and the gap between the second and first (or more accurately between the third and fourth) sounds is called diastole.

There have been numerous cases over the years of horses at the top of their particular field of athletic activity but whose proposed purchase has fallen through because a veterinary examination revealed a heart abnormality. These abnormalities may be of two types. They may be either heart murmurs, which are extra noises heard with the stethoscope, or arrythmias, when there is an irregularity of the normal heart rhythm. Heart murmurs are usually due to disorders in the flow of blood through the heart, owing, for example, to a lesion on one of the heart valves. It has been pointed out that not all obvious murmurs arise from significant lesions, and conversely not all significant lesions give rise to loud murmurs. By and large, murmurs occurring during diastole are more significant with regard to a horse's athletic performance than systolic murmurs. This is despite the fact that systolic murmurs are often louder when heard with a stethoscope, and are more common than diastolic murmurs. Abnormalities in the cardiac rythmn, especially if they persist or get worse as a result of exercise, tend to be more likely to interfere with a horse's athletic performance than heart murmurs.

The various activities of the heart are all regulated by electrical impulses. These spread out through the cardiac muscles and cause them to contract or relax, depending on which stage of the cycle has been reached. Relaxed cardiac muscle has a negative electrical charge. A process called depolarisation results in a flow of positive charges into the muscle cell. When it becomes positively charged, the cell contracts. The equine heart, just like that of human beings, has an automatic pacemaker, called the sinoatrial node, which is the originator of the process of depolarisation. These electrical changes in the heart muscle can be measured far away from the organ itself. This is the basis of electrocardiography, which is the measurement and visualisation of these electrical changes in the heart. Placing positive and negative electrodes

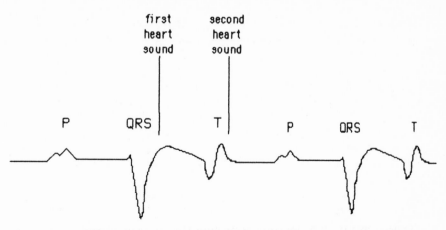

Fig 23 Electrocardiograph trace showing the letters used to identify the various features

in close contact with the horse's skin anywhere on its body will enable us to measure the electrical activity, but in order to give some order and meaning to what we find out, certain precise locations have been accepted for these electrodes. Fig 23 shows an electrocardiograph (ECG) trace. The ECG provides completely different information from the stethoscope. It is basically telling us about the electrical activity of the heart muscle cells.

The importance of the horse's heart rate

The horse's heart rate can vary so much that, depending on whether the horse is excited or not, there may be considerable uncertainty over what the normal resting heart rate of a particular horse actually is. The average resting heart rate of an adult horse is usually around 40 beats per minute. In extremely fit horses, however, resting heart rates as low as 24 beats per minute have been recorded. Exercise causes the heart rate to increase dramatically, so that when a horse is walking it will have a heart rate of around 80 beats per minute, when it is trotting the rate will increase to between 120 and 140 per minute, and when it reaches the canter the heart will be beating at around 160 and 200. A galloping horse will have a heart rate of over 200 beats per minute, and it may be as high as 250 beats per minute in young horses. It is very unusual for an animal the size of a horse to achieve such a high heart rate since, in general, the larger the species the lower the maximum heart rate which can be achieved. In man the maximum heart rate is just under 200 beats per minute, with resting rates of around 50 per minute. So the horse increases its heart rate almost tenfold with exercise, whereas man can only increase it fourfold.

Table 6 Approximate heart rates at different paces

	Beats/minute
Standing	40
Walking	80
Trotting (234m/min)	120
Trotting (298m/min)	140
Cantering (348m/min)	160
Cantering (500m/min)	200
Galloping (800–1000m/min)	200–250

Swimming can increase the heart rate to between 160 and 200 beats per minute. It follows that the use of swimming, either free or tethered, during a training programme (or during recovery from injury) must be good training for the oxygen circulating system, as well as keeping the muscles tuned. Tethered swimming puts a greater workload on the horse and so increases the heart rate more than free swimming.

When a horse is standing in the stable it is possible to measure its heart rate either by counting its pulse or by listening directly to its heart with a stethoscope. The horse's pulse is usually felt just on the inside of the lower jaw (Fig 24). It can take considerable practice to be able to feel a horse's pulse.

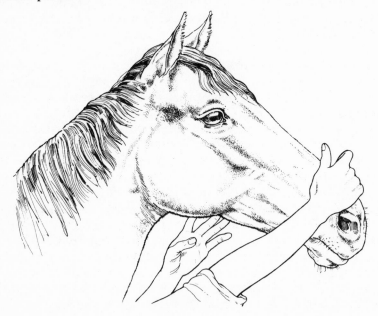

Fig 24 It is possible with the fingers to feel the facial artery under the skin as it passes around the lower edge of the lower jaw. Counting the pulsations of this artery provides the pulse rate

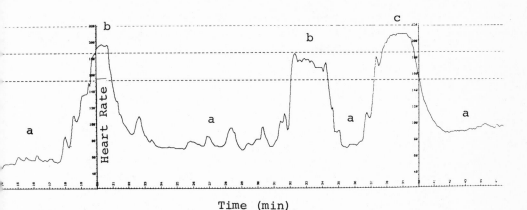

Time (min)

Fig 25 A heart rate trace obtained from an on-board heart rate meter (Hippocard – Ingenie-büro isler, Switzerland). The meter stores the information which then can be analysed on a computer and the required print out obtained. Stop watch facilities also allow different parts of the work period to be accurately timed. a-walk, b-canter, c-gallops.

The effects of exercise and disease on the heart

The fitter the horse is, the lower its heart rate at any particular speed of gait. For this reason, horse trainers have in recent years shown an interest in measuring their horses' heart rates to assess their fitness. Trainers are most concerned with what is happening to the horse's heart during movement, but it is obviously not possible to listen to this with an ordinary stethoscope. Recently, a number of cardiotachometers have become available (Plate 16) which give a digital readout of the heart rate at any particular moment. They might be considered to be very simple versions of the ECG, as they only count the number of complete cycles in a particular time. Although at moderate speeds these meters are easy to read, at fast gallops it becomes more difficult to read them, especially as the rider is also involved in steering the horse, etc. To overcome this problem, meters are available which allow the heart rate to be recorded and played back after the completion of the exercise (Fig 25). The heart-rate meters have electrodes in contact with the horse's skin, and the machine itself is attached to the rider, the saddle or the horse's neck. When the horse first moves off, there is a rapid rise in its heart rate, which then falls back to a plateau level after two or three minutes at that particular work rate. If, however, you take a horse more or less straight from a standing start into a flat-out gallop, this initial overshoot of the heart rate does not occur. Instead, the rate rapidly reaches the 'plateau' level. The overshoot in heart rate at slow paces is thought to be due to a delay in the horse mobilising the red blood cells

117

stored in its spleen. This is another reason why a warm-up period should be introduced before any strenuous exercise. Anticipatory stress, such as the excitement of horses being paraded around the ring prior to a race, will also help to prepare the heart because it leads to the release of adrenalin and the mobilisation of the red cells. Until these have been released, the horse needs more oxygen than it can obtain from the number of red blood cells circulating in its bloodstream, and so it has to pump them round more quickly in order to use each individual cell more often. Except at the very highest workloads, the horse's heart rate increases in direct proportion to its workload or speed of movement.

Just as the heart rate increases when the horse goes faster, so it decreases when the horse slows down. Fig 26 shows how the heart rate of a Standardbred trotter went up and down depending on the severity of the heats and race. It should also be noticed that the pre-race parade caused a marked rise in heart rate as the horse became excited. The time taken for the heart rate to return to each individual horse's resting rate after exercise is related to the intensity of the exercise and

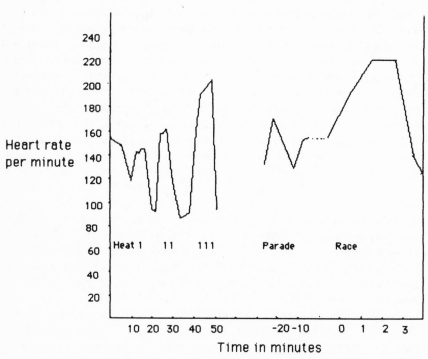

Fig 26 Trotter's heart rate before, during and after three heats and during a real race (Adapted from Asheim and others (1970) Journal of Am. Vet Med Assoc. *157*, 304-312)

to the fitness of the horse. The recovery is fastest in the fittest horses. It has been shown that the recovery in heart rate measured at thirty minutes after exercise is a reasonable indication of fitness because the results obtained fit in well with other measures of the horse's recovery from fatigue. This is used to determine the degree of fitness or fatigue during and after endurance rides.

Disease conditions, especially those affecting the respiratory system, will often affect heart rates. Horses suffering from chronic obstructive pulmonary disease (heaves) have been found to have heart rates twenty beats per minute higher during exercise than normal horses. The more severe the respiratory obstruction, the faster the heart rate. It has been possible, using radio transmitters attached to an ECG machine, to observe various abnormalities in ECGs during exercise. From the practical point of view, the most important point would seem to be that horses with abnormal ECGs tended to 'draw attention to themselves' by having higher than normal heart rates at exercise.

With the development of the various methods of investigating the structure and performance of the horse's heart, it is not surprising that researchers also began to look for ways in which the information which they could now obtain could be used either to assess fitness or to predict performance. It was obvious that the total cardiac output was important in any consideration of the heart's effect on performance. Cardiac output per minute is the heart stroke volume (the amount of blood pushed out of the heart with every beat) multiplied by the heart rate. In 1963 Steel in Australia devised a method for working out the approximate size of any individual horse's heart. The size of the heart is important because its stroke volume is regulated by the heart size. This heart size is, in turn, related to the volume of the heart ventricles. Obviously, the heart cannot have a stroke volume any greater than the ventricular volume, because the ventricle is the final chamber through which the blood passes before leaving the heart. It is certainly a fact that, in man, the very best athletes have large hearts. There is still some controversy, however, over the question of whether this is largely due to their genetic build, or to development of the heart muscles during training. When talking about a large heart, incidentally, we mean a heart which is large in relation to the body size of the individual, not just the large heart which is normal in a large body.

Steel devised a value which he called the heart score. This is obtained from ECG readings, and is defined as the arithmetic mean of the QRS interval (see Fig 23) obtained from each of three standard placings of the ECG electrodes. When the ECG tracing is printed out, it is possible to measure the time taken for each part of the trace. For the purpose of measuring a horse's score, the QRS intervals are measured to the nearest 10 milliseconds! A very good correlation has been found between heart score and the heart size (the actual correlation being 0.92). It is thus possible to say, for example, that a horse having a heart score of 100 will have a heart weighing 6.6lb (3kg), whereas a horse with a heart score of 130 will have a heart weighing 11.8lb (5.4kg). Mares and fillies generally have slightly lower heart scores than stallions and geldings, although it has to be pointed out that they also tend to have lower body-weights as well.

If heart scores are to have a relation to performance, it is in the longer distance activities that this is most likely to show, because a highly developed cardiovascular system is probably not so important in sprinters. This would seem to be borne out by the fact that a study of the major 'staying' handicap races in Australia (those over distances of 1½-2 miles (2,400-3,200m)) showed that they were generally won by horses with a heart score greater than 120. Other studies in standardbreds and in endurance horses have also shown that the better performers had the higher heart score. A study of heart score and performance in British flat-racers failed to find any effect of heart score on performance on the racetrack, but this study did not separate sprinters from stayers in their analysis.

Steel has even suggested that as heart size is a genetic factor, it should be possible to look at the heart score of yearlings and predict their future potential. The heart score will certainly be influenced by the horse's body-weight, and it is regrettable that so far no investigations have corrected the heart score for this factor. The results of the study of endurance horses previously mentioned, for instance, would have probably shown an even greater correlation between heart score and performance if this had been done because the horses were mostly Arabian or Arabian crosses which have a relatively low body-weight.

So far we do not know precisely what effect training has on the heart score. Training does, however, appear to result in a progressive increase in cardiac mass. This effect is age related in that over a certain age little further adaptation of heart size occurs despite further training. It may well be that the new technique of echo-cardiography will shed some new light on the effects of training on heart size. This uses beams of ultrasound similar to those used to scan pregnant women or mares. In this way it is possible to measure increases in ventricular wall thickness and in ventricular volume, information which cannot be obtained from an ECG. In human athletes it has already been shown that distance runners develop thicker ventricular walls than sprinters. There is every indication, therefore, that techniques such as heart score and echocardiography will eventually tell us more about a horse's potential for distance events, and its response to training for such events.

How blood flow and volume change with exercise
When a horse starts exercising, there is an almost instantaneous increase in the blood flow to the muscles which are working. This results from changes occurring within the contracting muscles, possibly involving the release of substances such as potassium. The capillary bed within the muscle then dilates. In the horse a seventy-fold increase in blood flow to active muscles has been reported, although in man it is more likely to be in the region of a fifteen-fold increase. In man, however, this increase has to be compensated for by a reduction in blood flow to non-exercising areas such as the intestines. This may not happen in the horse because it has a very large reservoir of red blood cells in its spleen which it can instantly utilise to increase the circulating blood volume. The increased blood flow to the muscles obviously results in their being able to take more oxygen out of the system, so that there is a greater difference between the concentration of oxygen in the arteries as the blood leaves the heart compared with the oxygen concentration in the veins bringing the blood back to the right side of the heart for reoxygenating in the lungs. During really strenuous exercise the horse can extract up to 90-95 per cent of the blood's oxygen content during its passage around the body. When the horse's muscles are working this hard they can develop areas of hypoxia, or oxygen shortage, because the forceful muscle contractions constrict the small arteries and so reduce the blood flow.

So far, we have been talking as if the cardiovascular system (the combination of the blood vessels, the heart and the blood which it pumps around the body) is dealing with a constant volume of blood. This is not the case. The horse's blood volume is determined by the amount of fluid, or plasma, and the number of cells in that plasma. Unlike in man, where there is a slight decrease in the circulating volume with exercise, when the horse is exercised its blood volume increases. This is because of the large number of red blood cells stored in the spleen of the resting horse. When the horse is excited in any way, whether it is just a stranger walking into its box or by having a good gallop, then without the horse consciously knowing that it is doing so, its sympathetic nervous system causes its spleen to contract. This system no doubt dates back to the days when the horse was wild on the plains and its reaction to fright was flight. So any fright causes an increase in circulating red blood cells, just in case extra capacity for oxygen transport should become necessary to the muscles of movement.

What is blood?

In any consideration of the athletic horse, it is obviously necessary to give some consideration to what blood is, how it changes during exercise, its possible role in the diagnosis of exercise-related problems, and more controversially, its potential as a source of information concerning assessment of fitness. The appeal of blood sampling in investigating such problems is obviously increased by the relative ease with which the samples can be taken. Unlike in man, blood samples in the horse are usually taken from the jugular vein, which runs along the lower part of the neck.

Blood consists essentially of two parts, the cells and the plasma. There are two kinds of cells, red blood cells (RBC) and white blood cells (WBC), and they each serve different functions. There are also cell fragments, called platelets, floating around in the plasma, and these are very important in aiding the rapid clotting of blood when bleeding occurs from a severed blood-vessel. Plasma consists largely of water, in which are dissolved thousands of different substances of varying molecular size. It contains:

1 Chemicals which are carried as nutrients to the various tissues of the horse's body.
2 Waste products which are transported from one tissue to another for disposal, eg to the liver or kidney.
3 Compounds involved in regulating cellular activity, ie hormones.
4 Substances involved in the defence of the horse's body against outside invaders.
5 Some substances which have leaked out of cells when temporary or permanent cell damage has occurred.

It is the measurement of changes in the levels of this latter type of chemical substance present in the blood which can be very important diagnostically in tracking down the site and extent of tissue damage in many clinical conditions.

The red blood cells

The red blood cells (RBCs) are also known as erythrocytes, and in the horse they are relatively small compared with other mammals such as man. This small size may possibly help in the loading and unloading of oxygen, as well as in their passage through the smallest blood-vessels, the capillaries. Unlike all other cells in the body, the red blood cells do not contain a nucleus, having lost this during their formation in the bone marrow. The major, and unique, component of the RBCs is a special protein called haemoglobin. This has a high content of iron, and its molecules occupy about one-third of the mass of all red cells. The func-

122

tion of haemoglobin is to transport oxygen from the lungs to the other tissues in the body so that it can be used to maintain aerobic metabolism. The normal oxygen-carrying capacity of haemoglobin is 1.34ml/g. The amount of haemoglobin present is obviously critical in determining how much oxygen can be transported to the tissues. Once it has unloaded its oxygen, the haemoglobin molecule can then help to remove the carbon dioxide formed during metabolism, because carbon dioxide can also become attached to the molecule. Generally speaking, haemoglobin picks up the gas which is in highest concentration (which is oxygen in the lungs, but is carbon dioxide in most other tissues) and releases it again when it reaches a tissue where there are low levels of the gas.

As has already been mentioned, the number of RBCs and the amount of haemoglobin can vary widely in the resting horse or pony. This may be due to genetic and physiological reasons as well as any effect owing to illness. The quantity of RBCs present can be expressed in a number of ways; as cells/ml, as haemoglobin g/l, or as an haematocrit. The latter is also known as the packed cell volume (PCV), and it is a measurement of the space in the blood volume which is occupied by the cells. Haematocrit is expressed as a percentage. So a horse with $9 \times 10_{12}$ cells will usually have a haemoglobin level of 150g/l and a haematocrit of 41 per cent.

Today's breeds have largely been evolved from two basic types of horse: the cold-blooded and the warm-blooded horses. These terms have nothing to do with the temperature of the blood, which is the same in both types. The latter are faster than the cold-blooded horses. In accordance with these evolutionary differences, it has been found that the number of RBCs in the circulation at rest may vary (Fig 27). Cold-blooded horses will have PCVs of 26-32 per cent, whereas in warm-blooded horses they will be 32-46 per cent. It is important for owners to realise this when blood samples are taken from their horses. Crossbreds obviously have intermediate values. Interestingly, it has been shown recently that by and large sprinting animals have lower haemoglobin levels and packed cell volumes than staying horses. In fact, some normal sprinters may have PCVs as low as 32 per cent, which could be considered a sign of anaemia, although this is not the case. As both groups of horses are thought to have similar values before entering training, the difference in PCV is considered to result from the different training regimes to which they have been subjected. The stayers undergo more aerobic work, which may act as a greater stimulus for the production of new red blood cells by the bone-marrow.

We have already mentioned that the number of red blood cells released into the general circulation from the horse's spleen is related to

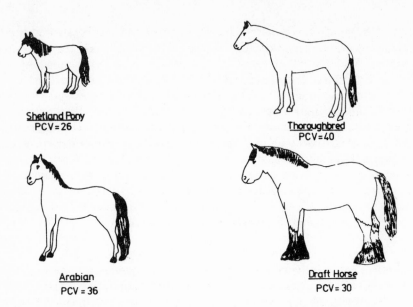

Shetland Pony
PCV = 26

Thoroughbred
PCV = 40

Arabian
PCV = 36

Draft Horse
PCV = 30

Fig 27 The resting packed cell volume (haematocrit) in different breeds

the intensity of the exercise which the horse is undergoing. Only small increases in PCV are seen at low speeds but there is complete splenic contraction at maximal speeds. In the thoroughbred and standardbred, haematocrits in excess of 65 per cent can occur during maximal effort. When this occurs, the oxygen-carrying capacity of the blood can increase from approximately 180ml at rest to 280ml of oxygen per litre of blood at exercise. This is one of the contributing factors to the very high maximal oxygen consumption levels which have been recorded in the horse. With this marked increase in circulating RBCs, there is an increase in viscosity, ie the blood becomes thicker. This raises the question of how long this type of 'thick' blood can be pumped around the circulation by the heart.

Although most of the increase in haematocrit is brought about by this influx of RBCs into the circulation, some of the change is due to the loss of water from the blood. This water moves into the surrounding tissues or is lost during sweating. Following maximal exercise it takes several hours before the haematocrit returns to normal pre-exercise values.

Because of the value of having a good supply of oxygen to tissues during exercise, it has been reported that some human athletes involved in long-distance races have resorted to artificially elevating their haematocrit prior to competing. This technique is called blood doping. It involves removing blood from the athlete some weeks prior to the competition, storing it either in a refrigerator or deep freeze, and then reinjecting it into the same athlete just before the race. By this time the original blood which was removed will have been replaced by fresh cells from the bone-marrow, so the reinfusion causes an increase in blood volume and hopefully also in performance. A similar ploy has been considered in the horse, and apparently also carried out, although its success has not been reported for obvious reasons. However, because of the horse's natural 'self-boosting' organ, the spleen, there appears to be no rational reason for using the technique in horses (Fig 28). It should also be pointed out that as certain compounds, known as anticoagulants, have to be used to preserve the RBCs during refrigeration, it is likely that attempts to use the technique could be detected where stringent drug detection procedures are being carried out.

Interpreting the red blood cell count

The usefulness or otherwise of taking resting blood samples from horses in order to try to assess their fitness and racing potential has been debated among exercise physiologists and veterinary surgeons for many

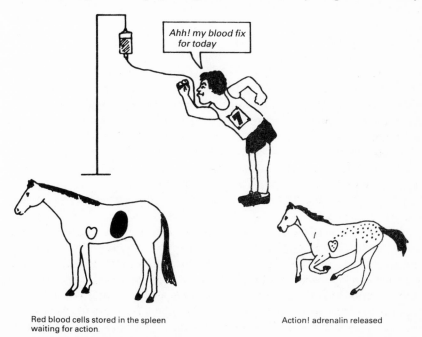

Red blood cells stored in the spleen waiting for action.

Action! adrenalin released

Fig 28 Although blood doping has been used in man to increase the amount of oxygen varied by the blood, this is unnecessary in the horse, as its spleen stores large numbers of red blood cells which are promptly released during exercise

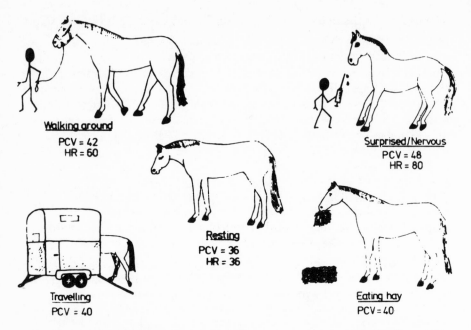

Walking around
PCV = 42
HR = 60

Surprised/Nervous
PCV = 48
HR = 80

Resting
PCV = 36
HR = 36

Travelling
PCV = 40

Eating hay
PCV = 40

Fig 29 A number of external factors can influence the resting packed cell volume. This makes the obtaining of resting values difficult

years. It has been suggested, for example, that horses with a low haematocrit or haemoglobin are likely to be less successful on the racetrack than those with higher values. There are, however, limitations to the value of such tests. First, as for so many tests, the value will depend on the quality of the sample obtained. For it to be of any possible use, the horse has to be in a truly resting state, free from the other factors which we have already said can cause false alterations in the haemotocrit. The factors which increase haematocrit are also those which result in the release of adrenalin (Fig 29). It is pointless, therefore, to collect samples from horses that become apprehensive or excited prior to collection, horses that have just been transported, or those which have just been exercised. In addition, factors which can alter the plasma volume can also cause false elevations of the haematocrit. These factors include the consumption of large quantities of hay immediately prior to sampling (Fig 29), and dehydration brought about by exercise or clinical illness, eg diarrhoea. A decrease in haematocrit can also be caused by the oral administration of salts to the horse, as is sometimes done on the day before racing. The problem associated with blood testing an apprehensive horse cannot be overcome by giving it a tranquilliser as most of these cause the spleen to take up RBCs and therefore give a falsely low haematocrit.

As has already been mentioned, there are genetic differences which account for variations in red blood cell values between breeds. It is likely that similar differences occur between different individuals within a breed. There are also variations with age. Younger horses, such as year lings and two-year-olds, have lower red blood cell values than older ones. The increasing values seen in older animals may result from either increasing maturity or from training effects (or possibly from both).

As it is the total number of red blood cells in the body that is of relevance to performance, rather than the number measured in the circulation of a resting horse, it would appear that the determination of the total blood volume, ie the volume after the spleen has been completely emptied, would be very useful. Total blood volume can be measured either after a period of maximal exercise or after the injection of adrenalin to empty the spleen. It is not just a low blood volume that suggests that there may be a problem either; a high blood volume may indicate that the horse has been 'overtrained'. Determination of the total blood volume is not a very popular test, possibly because it is more difficult to carry out than just obtaining a resting blood sample, but it should always be carried out if a problem is suspected relating to oxygen transport around the circulation. It is known that horses having different resting haematocrit levels may have a similar total blood volume and therefore similar oxygen-carrying capacities.

If resting blood samples are to be of any use, it is essential that they are always collected at the same time of day, eg in the morning prior to exercise and feeding or just before afternoon stables on a day of light work. One-off samples are of little use unless large variations are being looked for. Instead, samples should be collected at intervals during a training programme, with initial samples being taken before the training starts at all. In this way, conditions that might cause deviations for that particular animal can be pin-pointed. During the first year of training a general but moderate increase in red blood cell numbers, haemoglobin and haematocrit can be expected. Although a progressive increase in total blood haemoglobin associated with age has been demonstrated, the significance of any changes in red blood cell values after further time in training is debatable.

Anaemia is a term used to describe a decrease in the oxygen-carrying capacity of the blood below accepted normal levels. It can result from a reduction in either the total number of RBCs or in the haemoglobin content of the blood. Although anaemia is often given as an excuse for poor performance, all the evidence indicates that, in contrast to the situation in man, a true anaemia is very uncommon in the horse and so such a diagnosis is usually more imaginary than real. The important exception to this is that, in some parts of the world, infectious anaemias may occur, eg babesiosis or infectious viral anaemias. Anaemia, if it is present, can be brought about by three major causes:

1 Any cause of blood loss will cause a decrease in circulating red blood cells. Acute losses are seen following accidents causing haemmorhage, while the most common cause of chronic loss is parasitism. This latter cause should not be a problem in well-managed stables with good worming programmes, but unfortunately it is still a frequent occurrence in horses kept at pasture.

2 Destruction of red blood cells can obviously lead to a reduction in circulating RBCs. This is referred to as haemolytic anaemia, and may have various causes.

3 The most common cause of anaemia is a depression anaemia. It is generally seen in horses suffering from various diseases. The illness results in an increased lethargy in the animal, leading to reduced sympathetic nervous system activity (ie less adrenalin in the blood) and so to decreased activity in the bone-marrow which is quite secondary to the disease itself. As the animal throws off the primary condition, a return to the normal haematocrit occurs.

Obviously, if any of the causes of anaemia are present, veterinary attention for the animal is required to overcome the primary cause.

In parallel with imaginary anaemia, several myths have developed concerning the use of substances referred to as haematinics that are used to promote increased red blood cell formation. This has led to a plethora of preparations being available which are marketed with exaggerated and largely unsubstantiated claims as to their efficacy. The preparations can be given either in the feed or by injection and may contain one or more substances. Large amounts of money are spent on them by the equine industry and it is unlikely that one could visit a stable without seeing at least one of them in the feed room. They are frequently used without any veterinary approval or knowledge. Unfortunately, the little research that has been carried out on the use of these preparations does not substantiate the claims made for them. In contrast to man, it appears that only rarely are supplements containing iron or vitamin B_{12} required in horses as the horse normally has sufficient supplies of both. Another substance, folic acid, is of importance in red blood cell synthesis and it has been shown that stabled horses may have low blood levels of this substance. Unfortunately, it has also been found that only poor absorption of this substance occurs when it is given as a supplement in the feed despite the fact that it is naturally obtained from green feeds. Therefore, the best way of raising blood levels is by ensuring that adequate green feed, eg lucerne, is given on a regular basis.

The white blood cells

The other cells which are found in the cellular part of the horse's blood are the white cells (WBCs), or leucocytes. There are far fewer leucocytes in the blood than there are red blood cells – only about 8,000 million WBCs per litre of blood. When a blood sample is spun down in a centrifuge to allow the removal of the fluid plasma, the white blood cells form a very thin white layer above the red blood cells. Within this layer are several different types of WBC. Although each type of cell has a particular role to play, the white blood cells as a whole enable the horse's body to respond to, and hopefully resist, outside invaders such as viruses, bacteria and parasites. In addition, they are very important in the healing process of wounds and in other situations where inflammation occurs.

There are four major white blood cells: neutrophils, monocytes, eosinophils and lymphocytes (Plate 17). The first three of these cell types help the body get rid of any invading organisms, as well as any dying tissue around sites of inflammation. They achieve this either by engulfing the foreign material and digesting it, or by the release of chemicals which break down the material outside the leucocyte. The fourth type of leucocyte, the lymphocyte, is important because it produces the antibodies which help to immobilise outside invaders and foreign material. When there is a shortage of lymphocytes, the horse's ability to resist outside invaders is considerably reduced. It is also the lymphocytes that are largely responsible for the development of immunity following vaccination.

Looking at the leucocytes as a whole, the predominant cell type in the horse is usually the neutrophil. There are slightly fewer lymphocytes, and only small numbers of monocytes and eosinophils. During an infection, especially if it becomes generalised throughout the horse's body, a change is seen in the white cell picture, with an overall increase in total numbers occurring. Even in an acute infection, however, this increase is much smaller than that seen in man and most other animals. The extent of this increase in total WBC numbers, and the changes which occur in the individual cell types, help the veterinary surgeon to differentiate between various types of infection and also to monitor the progress of the condition. The total white blood cell count is slightly lower in older animals owing to a decrease in the numbers of circulating lymphocytes.

Interpreting the white cell count

Just as trainers and veterinary surgeons use the resting red cell values to help assess a horse's fitness, some have also placed their reliance on white blood cell counts. In particular, they have looked at the ratio of neutrophils to lymphocytes. In the truly fit and healthy racehorse, it is believed that there is an ideal neutrophil:lymphocyte ratio of around 60:40. Deviations from this may either indicate the presence of an underlying illness, even if this may not be clinically obvious, or it may indicate that the horse is under- or over-trained. Unfortunately, there is little scientific evidence either to back up this hypothesis or disprove it. Practical experience suggests that this ratio may indeed be useful, and that in many cases variations, especially when they reverse the ratio so that there are more lymphocytes than neutrophils, indicate that all is not well with the horse. It should be emphasised that at the present these comments are restricted to the Racing Thoroughbred. Just as is the case with RBC measurements, if any reliance is to be placed on total WBC counts, etc, it is important that the samples are taken from the horse at regular intervals during the training and racing season, so that the horse's normal base-line values can be established.

There is an optimal time for taking samples for WBC measurements, just as there is for RBC measurements. The total WBC count can also be affected by exercise. If a sample is collected immediately after maximal exercise, there might be a slight increase in total WBC numbers but, more importantly, further lymphocytes will have been added to the circulation and so the normal neutrophil:lymphocyte ratio may be reversed. It takes several hours of rest before the ratio returns to its base level. Following a prolonged period of exercise, the changes in WBC numbers become more marked as the release of neutrophils into the circulation causes an increase in total WBC numbers. This particular increase is the result of the release of a natural hormone called cortisol. It may take over twenty-four hours for a return to normal values, so there is little point in having a veterinary surgeon collect a blood sample within a day of prolonged exercise. Time and time again the trainers of beaten favourites in races have declared that they have had the horse blood tested on its return from the track and it had an abnormal blood cell count that indicated that it had an infection. If these samples are taken within twenty-four hours of the race, they are more likely just to indicate that the horse has had a race! This natural effect of cortisol is also important when considering the use of corticosteroids or ACTH to treat inflammatory conditions in the horse. An altered picture will be seen if samples are taken after the use of these compounds as well, and this has to be borne in mind when interpreting white cell counts on race-tracks where these drugs are frequently used.

The fluid component of the blood
The blood plasma or serum comprises the extracellular water of the

blood and thousands of different chemical substances which are carried in that fluid. These chemicals may have molecules which are very small in size, such as sodium, or they may be large and complex, such as proteins. The water of the plasma and the water of the interstitial fluid, the fluid which bathes the cells within the tissues of the body, intermingle through tiny pores in the blood capillary walls. These pores allow water and most dissolved substances, except proteins, to move freely between the plasma and interstitial fluid. The chemical substances dissolved in the plasma serve varying functions. Most of them are present because they are being transported from one tissue to another. It might be that they are needed as nutrients, or they might be waste products which have to be disposed of by the liver or kidney. The quantity of such substances present will vary according to the demands of the various tissues involved. For example, plasma glucose increases both at the start of exercise as it is mobilised from the liver, and after feeding as it is absorbed from the intestines. How the concentration of many of these substances changes during exercise gives us some insight into the metabolic demands of the exercise. As we can collect blood samples very readily, this provides a welcome research tool for exercise physiologists and biochemists. There are also some substances present in the plasma whose main role is to retain the water within the vascular system. If these were not present, all the water would flow out of the blood-vessels into the tissue spaces because of osmosis.

There are approximately 60g (just over 2oz) of proteins per litre of plasma. About half of this is found in the form of one protein called albumin. This has several important functions, including its ability to help transport smaller molecules, such as free fatty acids, around the body. The other major group of proteins is the globulins. These include the antibodies, and they play a vital role in the horse's ability to resist infection. A deficiency of some of these globulins makes the horse more susceptible to infection. On the other hand, there is an increase in the production of globulins during disease, and monitoring the type of change in levels which occurs helps the veterinary surgeon to obtain an insight into the type and stage of infection present.

Blood proteins and the fight against disease

The globulins are also affected by vaccination against disease. When some regulatory bodies in the UK, such as the Jockey Club, introduced compulsory vaccination against equine influenza, a number of trainers claimed that injecting such vaccines affected the performance of their horses. It is obviously very difficult to prove or disprove such a claim in relation to each individual horse's performance. To do so one would almost need to take daily blood samples and measure the antibody levels, etc before and after the vaccination and competition to show some association.

In the late 1970s, however, all the trotting horses born during one year in Sweden were given either equine influenza vaccine or some sort of placebo. None of the owners, trainers or veterinary surgeons were told which horses had received the vaccine and which ones had not. A very small number of side-effects were reported as being associated with the 'vaccination', but just as many horses which had not actually had any vaccine were reported as having side-effects as those which had been vaccinated. Close examination of these supposed side-effects of vaccination often showed that they were actually due to a true infection with one of the other respiratory disease viruses. The horses were then followed through their racing career, and it was found that vaccination did not have any detrimental effect on the number of races a horse entered, its race times or the amount of prize money it won. As the Swedish programme was a compulsory one on a nationwide basis, we can safely assume that no potential side-effect went unnoticed. It would appear, then, that vaccination programmes do not affect a horse's training and overall performance. Nevertheless, it is obviously desirable that every trainer has a basic knowledge of what is going on in the horse's bloodstream when a horse is vaccinated.

In addition to these major proteins, there are other proteins present in smaller quantities. Some of the hormones that are so important in regulating and co-ordinating the functions of cells in various parts of the body are proteins, eg insulin. Enzymes, which are involved as catalysts in reactions along the metabolic pathways, are also proteins, and they are found in varying concentrations in the plasma. As we will discuss shortly, the measurement of these enzymes in plasma is extremely useful in ascertaining sites of tissue damage.

During all types of exercise, as well as during diseases which produce dehydration, there is an increase in the concentration of proteins within the plasma. In neither of these situations is this increase due to new proteins entering the circulation; rather, it is due to water moving out, ie a reduction in plasma volume. During maximal exercise, such as sprinting, most of this water flows into the tissue spaces, but in long-term exercise it is completely lost from the body as sweat. In the latter case, water is also lost from the tissue spaces in an attempt to keep the water level in the plasma as high as possible in order to try to ensure adequate circulation to the muscles. When this water loss from the tissue spaces becomes marked, dehydration becomes discernible, as discussed elsewhere. Following endurance rides in adverse climatic conditions, water loss can become very marked, leading to plasma protein concentrations as high as 90g/l. Whereas there is a very rapid return of plasma volume following maximal exercise, due to regulatory mechanisms, after endurance rides it takes much longer because it is dependent on the further consumption of water before rehydration.

The role of plasma enzymes in diagnosing disease problems

Enzymes are proteins which catalyse reactions in metabolic pathways within tissues. As cells are continually being broken down and replaced, there is always a small release of enzymes into the plasma. This determines the normal base-line plasma enzyme activity. When tissue is damaged, however, the release of these enzymes into the plasma is markedly increased. For any particular enzyme, the extent of the increase is mainly dependent on the amount of tissue damaged, the concentration of the enzyme in the tissue, and on how rapidly the enzyme is removed from the plasma.

Some of the enzymes measured in plasma are considered to be non-specific, ie they are found in high quantities in all tissues, and therefore high levels only confirm that tissue damage is present somewhere in the horse's body. Other enzymes are considered fairly specific for certain tissues, and therefore are extremely useful in identifying the site of the tissue damage. There is an enzyme called aspartate aminotransferase (or AAT), for example. This enzyme, which used to be known as glutamic-oxaloacetic transferase (or GOT), is non-specific but is frequently measured for screening purposes. Creatine phosphokinase (or CPK), on the other hand, is considered very tissue specific for muscle in the horse and is useful in monitoring exertional rbabdomyolysis (tying-up or azoturia).

In equine veterinary practice, the main plasma enzymes monitored are as follows. For liver disease, gamma-glutamyl transpeptidase, sorbital dehydrogenase and lactate dehydrogenase are measured. For muscle damage, creatine phosphokinase and lactate dehydrogenase are determined, whereas for intestinal damage a specific form of alkaline phosphatase, referred to as intestinal alkaline phosphatase, is measured. To assess general tissue damage the enzymes aspartate aminotransferase and lactate dehydrogenase are monitored. In addition to being used to diagnose tissue damage, repeated measurement of plasma enzymes allows the time course of a disease to be investigated in order to see if recovery is taking place. The measurement of plasma enzyme levels can also be incorporated into a 'fitness profile' for competitive horses, as it is generally found that the racehorses who perform best have fairly constant enzyme levels. Fluctuations in creatine phosphokinase and aspartate aminotransferase may occur during training, especially when the horses are first introduced to hard work. This is probably due to slight damage being caused to muscle fibres that have not previously been used. In some racing animals it has been found that high activities of these particular enzymes can occur throughout the year. The reasons for this are obscure, as no obvious signs of muscle damage are present. These animals may be experiencing a less severe (or subclinical) form of azoturia, and therefore they should not be raced until the plasma enzyme levels are within the normal ranges.

Blood salts or electrolytes
Within the plasma are also found quantities of the various electrolytes which occur throughout the body. These electrolytes are also referred to as ions, as they are electrically charged. The positive ions are called cations, and the negative ones are called anions. The main electrolytes found in fairly large quantities are sodium, potassium, calcium, magnesium, chloride, phosphate and bicarbonate. The first four of these are positively and the last three negatively charged. They are also often referred to as salts. In addition, other chemical elements such as iron, copper, manganese, selenium, zinc, cobalt, sulphur and iodine are also found within cells in small, or trace, amounts. When an excess or a deficiency of one of the electrolytes is suspected, the general status of the electrolyte in the horse's body is generally assessed by measuring its plasma concentration. However, this may only be of assistance in detecting very marked changes.

The major electrolytes are vital in maintaining the integrity of the physiological and biochemical processes within the cells. Alterations in their concentrations within the body can upset delicate balances and may impair performance or lead to clinical disease. Sodium is the major electrolyte in the interstitial fluids surrounding the cells, as well as in the plasma. Potassium is the major electrolyte within the cells. By having these different cations inside and outside the cell, an 'electrolytic gradient' is established which is important for triggering off the electrical activity necessary for the normal working of nerve and muscle cells. The respective roles of these electrolytes have developed from the evolution of early prehistoric life from the seas, when single cells were surrounded by sea water high in sodium and chloride. Much smaller amounts of calcium and magnesium are found in the blood and cells.

As far as the negatively charged electrolytes are concerned, chloride is found in the highest quantities outside the cells.Its main role is to help to balance the positive charge of sodium. Phosphate is another important anion as it is involved in combination with numerous compounds in metabolic and synthetic pathways. Bicarbonate is also important as it is part of what is referred to as the buffering system of the body. In other words, it helps to maintain the normal neutral environment of the body when chemical processes occur that may increase its acidity or alkalinity. For example, during maximal exercise lactic acid is produced, together with large numbers of hydrogen ions. If these hydrogen ions cannot be neutralised, acidity of the body occurs, as discussed elsewhere. Bicarbonate helps in the important neutralisation process.

With exercise there are shifts of the electrolytes between the cells and the blood. There may therefore be a slight increase in the plasma concentration of potassium, calcium and phosphate. With maximal exercise there is, on the other hand, a marked decrease in bicarbonate. During prolonged exercise, other changes occur as the electrolytes are lost in the sweat. It is generally only in these circumstances that electrolyte changes lead to problems. Usually, these shifts are quickly reversed at the completion of the exercise. Where, however, sweating has been pronounced, it may be advisable to give extra electrolytes in the horse's drinking water.

It is possible with intensive training, especially in climates where horses often sweat profusely, for high losses of certain electrolytes, especially sodium, to occur. These losses may not be completely replaced from the horse's normal diet. In these circumstances there may be an impairment of the horse's normal performance as well as, in more severe states, obvious clinical signs. Unfortunately, a deficiency of these electrolytes cannot readily be detected. The plasma concentration is often normal because the horse's homeostatic, or self-regulatory, mechanisms maintain the plasma levels at the expense of tissue levels. For a veterinary surgeon, therefore, to diagnose the less severe electrolyte disturbances that may result from overwork and/or incorrect feeding, he will need to take both a blood and a urine sample. Provided these samples are obtained within a relatively short time of each other, an indication can then be obtained of the balance of electrolytes within the body. Where abnormalities are found, an attempt can then be made to correct them.

6 · The Respiratory System

In the preceding chapters the necessity for a supply of oxygen for the continual generation of energy for cells to function has been described. We have also shown how, in the horse, muscle can dramatically increase its utilisation of oxygen and how this need is met by the ability of the cardiovascular system to vastly increase its oxygen delivery to the tissues. Obviously, all these changes could not occur if oxygen was not able to enter the body in sufficient quantities. It is the purpose of the airways and lungs to transfer oxygen from the air, normally containing 20.9 per cent of this life-giving gas, to the internal milieu of the body. These structures are usually described as forming the respiratory system; the airways from the nostrils to the entrance of the chest cavity is the upper portion, and that within the chest the lower. In addition to its vital role in transferring oxygen to within the body, the respiratory system is also involved in the removal of the waste carbon dioxide which has been formed in the mitochondria and also some of the excess water. Strictly speaking, the respiratory system can also be considered to cover all those structures involved in the processes of the transport of oxygen to the tissues, its passage into cells and its utilisation within the mitochondria (Fig 30).

Plate 9 Muscle fibres cut very thinly in cross section and stained to identify contractile (speed) characteristics. (*left*) Type I = slow contracting (twitch) fibre. Type II = fast contracting (twitch) fibre. (*right*) Using different staining conditions Type II fibres can be divided into A & B sub groups

Plate 10 Muscle fibres can also be distinguished according to their capacity to use oxygen. The dark and intermediate stained fibres have a high to moderate capacity for oxygen. The palest staining, generally the largest fibres have a low ability to use oxygen. These are Type II B fibres, and are only used at the fastest speeds

Plate 11 Schematic illustrations of the recruitment of muscle fibres at different intensities of exercise. O = fibres recruited at walk, O+ + recruited at moderate trot, O+ +* = at fast canter, O+ +*+ = at gallop. Note that as speed increases more and more fibres contract so that sufficient power can be generated. In this not fully trained animal, increases in speed result in low oxidative fibres being recruited at the canter and trot. These fibres will rapidly build up lactate and become fatigued

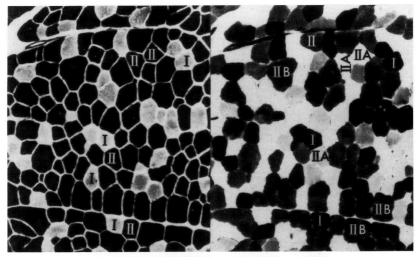

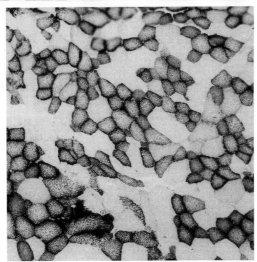

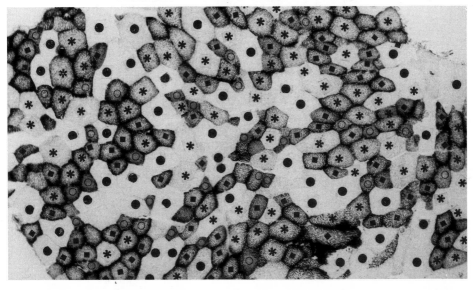

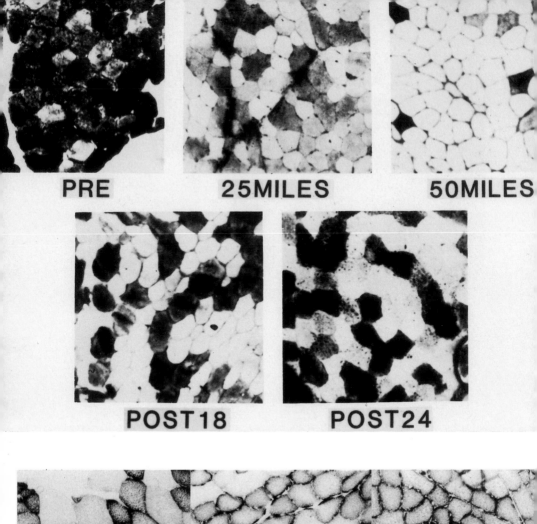

PRE   25MILES   50MILES

POST18   POST24

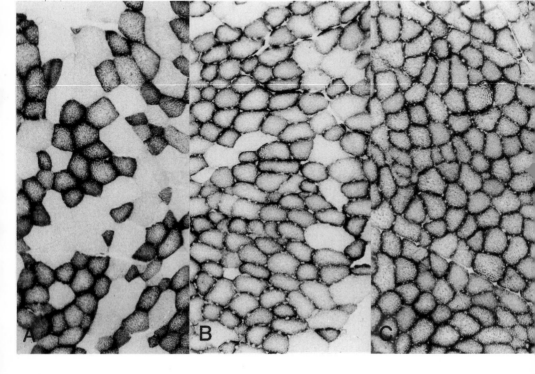

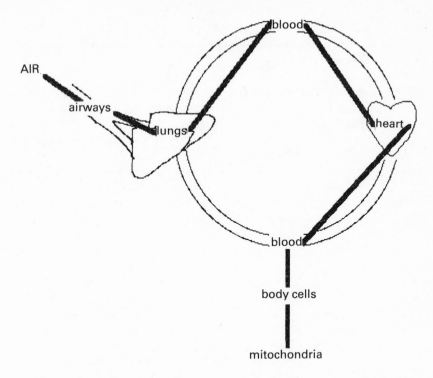

Fig 30 Oxygen transport from the atmosphere to the cells in the horse's body

The effective transport of oxygen into the body is dependent on three important processes: ventilation, diffusion and perfusion. Ventilation refers to the bulk movement of air into and out of the lungs. Diffusion is the term used to describe the passage of gases across the membranes separating the external environment, within the lumen of the millions of small sacs in the lungs, and the blood in the capillaries. Perfusion refers to the supply of blood to the capillaries surrounding these tiny sacs or gas exchangers known as alveoli. All of these three processes increase with exercise to ensure that the oxygen demands of the tissues are met.

Within this chapter, not only will the structures of the respiratory system and their functioning be outlined, but also attention will be given to

Plate 12 In prolonged exercise fatigue results from glycogen depletion. The darker the fibre the more glycogen it has. Note the slow repletion of glycogen stores following exercise (post 18 and 24 hours)

Plate 13 Improvement with training in the proportion of high oxidative fibres. A) early training, B) late training, C) after 2 years training

,the numerous conditions that can affect this system, hampering gas exchange and thus contributing to a reduced exercise tolerance especially at the higher workloads.

The upper respiratory system

All the air the horse takes into the lungs has to come via the nostrils, each of which is only about $2\frac{1}{4}$in (6cm) in diameter. Therefore, during exercise these have to work under considerable pressure, especially as the external inlets, the nostrils, can be distended by flaring. This sole reliance on the nostrils for air intake is in contrast to man, where the volume of air inhaled can be increased by mouth breathing. This inability to mouth breathe is because in the horse the air and food are kept completely separate. Whereas in human beings the pharynx is a joint chamber at the back of the mouth, with entrances from both the nostrils and the mouth and exits both to the larynx, or voice-box, and the oesophagus, in the horse this is not the case. Its pharynx is divided completely into two by the soft palate. The entrance to the larynx fits through this soft palate rather like a collar stud fits through its hole in the shirt. This arrangement allows air to pass into the larynx and down to the lungs without hindrance. When the horse swallows food, the larynx is completely closed off by a flexible flap of cartilage, the epiglottis, so that there is no danger of the food entering the lungs (Fig 31). A side-effect of this system is that, as has been mentioned, air coming in through the horse's mouth cannot get up through the hole in the soft palate and into the larynx and lungs.

There is one exception to this situation which can cause problems for the athletic horse. In a few horses, when they are literally at the limits of their performance and are desperate for oxygen, the muscles down the neck will pull the larynx out of its position in the soft palate. The horse then makes a gurgling sound and slows down extremely quickly because it is no longer getting a proper air supply. When this happens, the horse is often said to have swallowed its tongue, although, as will be appreciated, the tongue has not really been responsible for it at all.

The traditional way of dealing with such horses is to apply a tongue strap. This holds the tongue firmly to the bottom jaw and prevents it from being pulled backwards in the mouth. Because the muscles which pull the larynx out of its socket are also the ones which pull the tongue backwards, tying the tongue down in this way may stop the problem. Unfortunately, to be effective the tongue strap has to be fastened very tightly. It must not be left in place for long periods as it will cut off the circulation to the tongue. In recent years, a surgical treatment called myectomy has been developed. This consists of cutting the so-called

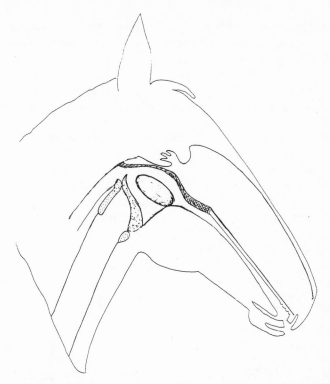

Fig 31 A cross section of the horse's larynx and pharynx during swallowing. The cross-hatched area shows the soft palate raised to block off the back of the nose (so that food does not escape down the nostrils). The stippled area shows the epiglottis sealing the entrance to the larynx (so that food does not get down the treachea into the lungs). The food is shown as a solid "bolus" (Courtesy T. Greet)

'strap' muscles down the horse's neck. The gap which is left is healed with scar tissue, and this effectively strengthens the muscles. As a result, they do not develop such tension when the horse is at the limits of its performance and dislocate the larynx so disastrously. Unfortunately this operation is not always successful in overcoming the problem.

Between the nostrils and the pharynx the air passes over the turbinate bones. These are thin plates of bone which are covered with a mucous membrane which is very rich in blood-vessels. Each side of the horse's face has both a dorsal and ventral turbinate bone. The bone plates are rolled up, rather like a scroll or a Swiss roll without any filling. Their purpose is to warm up the air which is entering the respiratory system so that cold air does not come into contact with the delicate membranes further down. If it did so, it would not only inhibit their resistance to infection, etc, but would also reduce the efficiency of the transfer of gases into the bloodstream and reduce blood flow through the lungs. If horses are subjected to training at fast speeds when the atmospheric temperature is too low, the turbinate system may not be able to warm up the air sufficiently, and problems may still occur. Special face masks are available for horses exercising in very cold climates which reinforce the effect of the turbinate bones by causing microturbulence of the air before it ever gets into the nostril. As turbulence warms up the air, this usually solves the problem. The scroll-like structure of the turbinates also helps to trap dust particles suspended in the air which is breathed in. The nasal passages humidify the inspired air so that it is fully saturated with water before it enters the lungs. This is achieved by having the cells lining the nasal passages (the nasal mucous membrane) secrete a clear watery fluid which keeps the surface of the membrane permanently moistened. The two functions of warming and humidifying help to ensure that a gas mixture of constant temperature and humidity is brought into contact with the delicate lining of the alveoli in the lungs. The aim is to provide a constant environment for the exchange of gases such as oxygen under a wide range of climates and fitness states.

The larynx is a cartilaginous tube. In the roof on either side of the passage-way are two cartilages called the arytenoid cartilages. Fibrous cords run from the bottom of the arytenoid cartilages to the floor of the passage-way and these support two folds of mucous membrane which make up the vocal cords (Fig 32). Between each vocal cord and the wall of the larynx is a saccule of mucous membrane which is rather like a balloon before it has been blown up. These are called the ventricles. Originally, we only knew of these structures from dissections of dead horses, but by using an instrument called a flexible endoscope it is now possible to examine the living horse's respiratory tract as far as the larynx, and even beyond (Plate 18). The vocal cords act rather like curtains across the airway through the larynx. When the horse is at rest or only moving slowly, they hang inwards, but when the horse needs more air for strenuous exercise, muscles pull the arytenoid cartilages outwards and so open the curtains to allow more air through without hindrance.

The larynx is another site where turbulence occurs. In all horses the air-flow out through the larynx during the canter and the gallop becomes so turbulent that it makes a noise. As the horse breathes out at the same time as the leading leg hits the ground (for reasons which will be discussed later), all horses make a noise on expiration at these gaits. In fact, work with radio stethoscopes attached to galloping horses has shown that even in normal horses there is some noise at inspiration. We do not usually hear this noise because it is no more than half the volume of that made at expiration. In many horses a whistling noise can be heard on inspiration at the canter if we listen carefully enough, although the noise may not occur all of the time. In a few horses, a distinct roaring noise can be heard at this time. The radio stethoscope shows that these horses are making just as much noise at inspiration as they are at expiration.

The problem of a 'roarer'

A 'whistler', a horse which makes a whistling noise on inspiration at the canter, does so because the left laryngeal ventricle is open and is acting as a resonance chamber. This happens because of a slight flaccidity of the left vocal cord. It appears that the left recurrent laryngeal nerve, the nerve which activates the muscles controlling the movement of the left arytenoid cartilage, tends to degenerate and so does not control the left vocal cords as well as that on the right. A 'roarer', or a horse which makes a roaring sound on inspiration at the canter, does so because the left vocal cord is not pulled out of the way of the increased air-flow (Fig 32). This condition is called laryngeal paralysis or laryngeal hemiplegia. Naturally occurring laryngeal hemiplegia always affects the left side of the larynx. The left recurrent laryngeal nerve is longer than the nerve on the right side. Incredible as it may seem for nerves which control a part of the body right up in the throat region, they start deep down in the horse's thorax. Whereas the right recurrent laryngeal nerve has a comparatively direct route up the neck to the larynx, the nerve on the left side first of all loops even further away, around the base of the major artery of the body, the aorta, before coming forward to the neck. Presumably, it is this extra length of the left nerve, coupled with the stretching which it might receive from the pulsing of the aorta, which makes it so prone to degeneration.

As all the air for the horse's lungs must pass through the comparatively narrow opening of the larynx, it is natural to assume that any defect of the larynx will have a serious effect on the oxygen supply to the horse. If the air-flow was smooth and without turbulence, this might well be the case. As it is, the air reaching the larynx already has a certain degree of turbulence from its passage through the nasal passages and over the turbinate bones, and this makes a significant difference to the situation. It has been shown that up to 40 per cent of the airway can be obstructed at the larynx before it significantly increases resistance to air-flow. This means that laryngeal hemiplegia may not affect a horse's performance at all unless it reduces the cross-sectional area of the airway through the larynx by more than 40 per cent. This supports what some veterinary surgeons have been saying for some time, namely, that many 'roarers' can perform normally as long as the trainer gets them properly fit. The tendency is, however, for the trainer not to exert the horse once they hear the noice, and so the horse does not receive normal training, and consequently does not perform as well as it could do.

There seems no reason for making the presence or absence of a noise at inspiration the final arbiter of whether a horse can perform up to its maximum potential or not. After all, there are many horses which make such a noise, but do not have any laryngeal abnormality at all. Swelling of the areas of lymphoid tissue in the roof of the pharynx, which trap infections, etc, can make a horse 'roar', for example. At present, we have the ridiculous situation where the major Thoroughbred sales yard in the

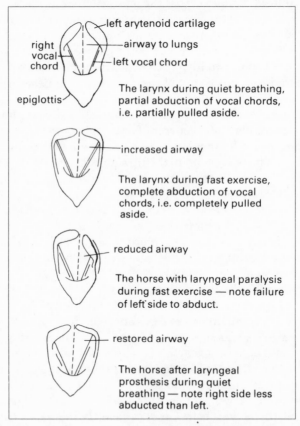

Fig 32 A) the larynx during quiet breathing, partial abduction of vocal chords, i.e. partially pulled aside. B) the larynx during fast exercise, complete abduction of vocal chords, i.e. completely pulled aside. C) the horse with laryngeal paralysis during fast exercise – note failure of left side to abduct. D) the horse after laryngeal prosthesis during quiet breathing

UK declares that a yearling cannot be returned as unsuitable even if it has complete paralysis of the left vocal cord until it also makes a roaring noise! This sort of attitude may well stem from the fact that the surgical procedure most commonly carried out to correct the condition of roaring, does more to reduce the noise than it does to increase the airway.

This traditional form of surgery is the so-called Hobday operation (although it was a gentleman called Williams who actually devised it and not Professor Hobday at all). It consists of removing the membranous linings of the laryngeal ventricles. The expectation is that when the resultant hole heals with scar tissue, the scar will pull the vocal cords outwards and so correct the fault. Since the advent of the endoscope it has become apparent that, in the vast majority of cases, this just does not occur. Most horses have the same cross-sectional area for air-flow through the larynx after the operation as they did before it. It is true that many horses make less of a roaring noise after the operation than they did before, although the precise benefit that this presumed decrease in turbulence brings, is hard to define. Professor Hobday, incidentally, who did so much to popularise the operation and who probably carried out more of these operations than anyone else, claimed that only 20 per cent of his cases reduced the noise sufficiently to appear cured to the 'average hunting man'. More recently, a new operation has been developed specifically to enlarge the airway in horses with laryngeal hemiplegia. This is the laryngeal prosthesis operation. It involves using an elastic thread, such as lycra, to tie the left arytenoid cartilage out in the normal galloping position. This is a much more intricate operation but does have the merit of doing what the horse owner expects it to do, namely, allow a normal amount of air down into the horse's lungs.

Having passed through the larynx, the air continues down the trachea, or wind-pipe, and then enters the chest cavity. Within the chest cavity the trachea divides into bronchi which then keep branching into progressively smaller tubes as the air is carried to all parts of the lungs. The trachea and bronchi are able to form flexible but non-collapsible tubes due to cartilaginous rings in their walls. Lining the inner surface of these airways are special cells which not only secrete the watery tracheal-bronchial mucus, but may also possess minute hair-like projections, called cilia (Plate 19). The function of the mucus is to keep the lining cells moist as air passing over them at high flow rates would otherwise quickly dehydrate them. The cilia, by beating in a co-ordinated pattern, act as an escalator to carry the mucus and foreign particles, such as dust, bacteria and fungal spores, up towards the larynx. There they are swallowed, coughed out or allowed to drain out as a nasal discharge. Therefore, these parts of the respiratory tract act as a highly efficient air cleaner, without which the alveoli would rapidly become overwhelmed with potentially dangerous material.

The problems associated with dust in the stables

The air which our horses breathe is even more dust-laden than that which we breathe because they are often bedded on dusty straw and spend hours with their noses buried in nets of dusty hay. Thankfully, the larger solid particles do not penetrate all the way down to the alveoli. They 'sediment' out in the turbinates and the larger airways such as the trachea or the bronchi, but some of the smaller particles are carried all the way down every time the horse breathes in. Activities such as mucking out the stable or filling the hay net dramatically increase the number of dust particles in the air. Poor ventilation reduces the rate at which these particles are then removed from the stable. It therefore follows that, whenever possible, mucking out should be carried out while the horse is out of the stable. It is better to get the stable bed ready before exercising the horse, as this gives time for the dust particles to settle before the horse is reintroduced into the atmosphere. The temptation to shut all the doors and windows during cold weather in order to protect the so-called sensitive competition horse should also be resisted.

As far as the horse's body is concerned, dust particles are foreign bodies and there is a specific procedure which is followed whenever foreign bodies gain access to the body. It is true that the particles are not actually inside the body in many ways, but the distance between the air and the blood cells in the alveoli is, as has been mentioned, very small. All horses therefore show a foreign body response to dust particles in their lungs. Whether this constitutes a problem or not will depend on many factors, of which the most important would appear to be how many particles are present in the air and for what length of time they are present.

In some horses, the natural defence mechanisms against these foreign bodies go haywire and the lungs become hypersensitive to one or more of the types of particles which are present. The most common particles to be involved in this hypersensitivity are fungal spores of the *Micropolyspora and Aspergillus* families. These fungae are almost invariably present on hay and straw, and it has been estimated that there may be as many as 16 million spores in each breath a horse takes. It must be stressed that most hypersensitive horses are allergic to the fungae, etc, and not to dust. It is true that such horses may be generally more sensitive to other irritants, such as the dust from clipping horses, and they may also respond more readily to respiratory infections, but these are not the underlying causes of the problem.

In the lungs themselves, the problem is triggered off by the neutrophils releasing cell toxins, enzymes and mediators. In addition cells called mast cells are involved. These contain substances such as histamine which, if they escape, will cause constriction of the tiny airways, increased mucus production and other signs of inflammation. The hypersensitive horse has more mast cells than normal in its lungs and their cell walls are more fragile. Consequently, they break open easily and release these chemicals into the lung tissue. The result is Chronic Obstructive Pulmonary Disease (COPD) (heaves or broken wind), because the bronchoconstriction, excess mucus and inflammatory thickening of the airway walls, causes narrowing of the airways and consequently obstruction of the airflow into the alveoli.

COPD horses have a chronic cough as they try to clear the thick mucus from their lungs. They may well also have a nasal discharge as a result of the cilia in the respiratory system bringing some of this mucus up to the pharynx. As the condition worsens, the horse will breathe more quickly even at rest and may show a characteristic heaving while doing so. This is because the normal elasticity of the lungs is no longer sufficient to empty them, and the horse has to use the muscles of the chest and abdomen to physically empty the lungs at each breath. This often results in the development of a 'heave line' along the sides of the abdomen where the muscles have been abnormally developed by extra use.

Treatment of COPD must first of all concentrate on removing the thing to which the horse is hypersensitive. Ideally, this will involve keeping the horse entirely outside so that it gets the maximum amount of fresh air. If this is not possible and the horse must be stabled, then it should be kept on some bedding other than straw, eg wood shavings, peat, or shredded paper. Even so, care must be taken not to allow these beddings to become sodden with urine as in such circumstances they, too, may harbour the dreaded fungae. The fresh air approach must apply to the whole air space involved. It is no use bedding one horse on shavings if the horse on the other side of some railings is on straw; the spores will soon get into the lungs of the COPD horse. There are two types of drug therapy similar to that used in human asthmatics available for such horses. Bronchodilator drugs, of which clenbuterol (Ventipulmin) appears to be the most successful in the horse, stimulate the muscles which open the bronchioles, and so reverse the action of histamine, etc. Sodium cromoglycate (Cromovet), on the other hand, acts to protect the mast cell walls so that they are less prone to rupture, and so less histamine is released.

Once a horse develops an allergy, that allergy will remain for the rest of its life. In fact, repeated exposure to the allergen, in this case the fungal spores, will result in the horse becoming more and more sensitive. Horses may become desensitised either by natural exposure or by heavy doses of the allergen. What remains for the rest of its life is the structural damage to lung tissue. The classic picture that develops is that the horse starts to cough a little towards the end of the stabling period for competition. This cough disappears when the horse is turned out for a rest. When it is brought back inside for the next season's competition, the cough appears even sooner. Eventually, the horse may show symptoms within days or even hours of being brought into a contaminated air space. It is important to realise that, as far as the athletic horse is concerned, the cough is not the important part of the problem. The bronchoconstriction is the symptom which effects the horse's performance. In the early stages, a horse may have loss of performance as a result of bronchoconstriction without a noticeable cough. Where there is any doubt about whether a horse has slight COPD or not, it is possible to give an intravenous injection of a bronchodilator and note any alteration in its breathing or performance. It would appear that widespread obstruction of the small airways, such as occurs in COPD, is critical for a horse's performance, and is certainly more important than obstruction of the upper airways, such as occurs in laryngeal hemiplegia, even though the latter is more dramatic to the lay onlooker.

The lungs

As already described, air is carried through the spongy lung tissue by tubes of progressively decreasing size with the final ones only being a fraction of a millimetre in diameter and without any supporting cartilage. These tubes end in a cluster of tiny air sacs, the alveoli, where gas transfer occurs. At this level the membranes lining the alveoli are very thin, being only one cell thick. This allows oxygen to pass from the alveoli through the wall of the capillaries (also one cell thick) surrounding the alveoli into the blood. Carbon dioxide is transferred in the opposite direction. The thin walled alveoli are prevented from collapsing by the production of a unique substance, called lung surfactant. As already stated, this process of transfer of gases is referred to as diffusion, and the force that drives it is the difference in partial pressure of the gases between the alveolus and the capillary blood. A gas flows from an area of high partial pressure to one of low pressure. Thus, diffusion is not only responsible for the movement of gases in the lungs, but also elsewhere in the body, eg working muscle. The approximate partial pressures of oxygen and carbon dioxide at various sites in the body is shown in Table 7.

Table 7   Amounts of oxygen and carbon dioxide present in the air and various body tissues

The partial pressures of oxygen and carbon dioxide are measured in millimetres of mercury

Tissue	Oxygen	Carbon dioxide
Atmosphere	160	0.05
Lung alveoli	149	40
Pulmonary veins	100	40
Large arteries	100	40
Capillaries	30–60	40–48
Muscle cells	10–30	50–80
Veins	40	46

For its body-weight, the horse has a relatively large lung (also known as pulmonary tissue) allowing a large surface area for diffusion. It has been estimated that if the pulmonary tissue of an adult Thoroughbred was spread out as one single sheet of tissue, it would cover an area of more than 1,200sq yd (1,000sq m). To allow the lungs to expand fourfold during breathing, the lung contains a great deal of elastic tissue, so much, in fact, that it contains even more per unit mass than the tendons which are always thought of as being so powerfully elastic in their function.

In addition to providing a mechanism for exchanging gases, the lung tissue has to manufacture the lung surfactant which has already been mentioned, provide cells (macrophages) to act as roving scavengers engulfing bacteria, etc, and also manufacture certain important enzymes. All in all, the horse's lungs comprise a complicated but vital system. It is not, however, a system in isolation. The lungs are, for example, the only organ through which the entire output of the heart passes. Venous blood is pumped through the lungs by the right ventricle of the heart. Within the fraction of a second (less than 0.2 seconds) during which each red cell is passing through the capillaries in the alveolar walls, its haemoglobin becomes saturated with oxygen and gives up its carbon dioxide. In little more than half a minute the entire blood supply of an adult Thoroughbred passes through the lungs. There are no significant short circuits; all the blood has to flow through capillaries which are only a fraction wider than the diameter of a red blood cell. The lungs therefore also act as a built-in filter for the blood. Foreign particles such as bacteria, cell fragments, small blood clots and other debris become trapped in the arterioles, or very small arteries, where macrophages and other scavenger cells deal with them. The large veins of the blood circulation in the lungs also act as a reservoir of blood which can be rapidly mobilised in times of stress.

During exercise, the blood flow or perfusion of the lungs can be markedly increased in order to match the increased cardiac output and oxygen requirements of the body. Just as in muscle, this occurs largely by the opening up of previously closed capillaries surrounding the alveoli. Recently, it has been found that at high workloads in Thoroughbreds and Standardbreds complete saturation of haemoglobin as it passes through the lungs does not occur, and therefore oxygen delivery is not as great as might be expected. This might also point to the lungs as being a limiting factor at very high workloads. The reason for this incomplete loading of the haemoglobin is presently unknown, but may be due to the very rapid passage of blood through the alveolar beds. Interestingly, a similar phenomenon has not been shown in ponies.

From the description of how gases pass to or from the internal to the external environment, it can be appreciated that anything causing damage to the lungs will impair diffusion. A number of infectious agents or other materials inhaled will establish an inflammatory response that can lead to the laying down of extra tissue around the alveoli which will disturb normal diffusion. Normally, such damage only involves a small portion of the lungs – and therefore normal respiration can occur at rest and even light exercise. However, with heavy exercise in which the full reserves of the lungs are required, it is apparent that any tissue damage will reduce the reserves available. Although as yet not studied, this is likely to cause even further desaturation of the haemoglobin. Therefore, it is little wonder that even minor damage can cause a dramatic reduction in performance. Such impairment may account for the rapid fading of horses seen on the racecourse, despite satisfactory training gallops. In races all the reserves are called upon, while during training, when only three-quarter speeds are required, full capacity is not necessary. Although viral infections are thought to be a common cause of this loss in performance, it is more likely that secondary bacterial infections will cause some lung damage with the effects described above.

The control of breathing
Ventilation, or the movement of air into and out of the lungs, consists of inhalation (inspiration) and exhalation (expiration) and is regulated by three factors. The first two are important at the walk and trot, while the third operates at the canter and gallop. First, it is controlled by chemical factors. The amounts of oxygen and carbon dioxide dissolved in the blood at any one time are constantly being monitored by sensors in the body. If the level of carbon dioxide in particular gets too high, then the message will be passed via the respiratory centre in the brain to increase the ventilation of the lung. This is achieved by breathing more deeply, if the

horse is not already using all its lung capacity, and by breathing more frequently. There is also a nervous control of ventilation. Because the horse naturally responds to a threat by flight, at the first sign of danger it will speed up its rate of breathing so that its blood and tissue oxygen levels start off as high as possible. A nervous horse will respond to the slightest disturbance by an increase in heart and respiratory rate. The third form of control is a mechanical one by which the respiratory rate is linked to the way in which the horse is moving.

The muscles which expand the rib-cage also tend to rotate the front legs forwards. At the walk and the trot this does not matter very much because the respiratory rate is not too fast, and the depth of ventilation is not too great. In any case, at these gaits, as discussed earlier, the legs on opposite sides of the horse's body are moving alternately. At the canter and gallop, however, the two legs are basically moving forwards together.

This synchronisation, coupled with the need for maximum chest expansion at these gaits, leads to the leg and chest movements becoming inextricably linked together. At the canter and gallop, the stride rate equals the respiratory rate (Fig 33). This is referred to as locomotory-respiratory coupling and is considered to be mechanically advantageous, as muscles do not have to work against each other. This process may also explain why the horse is able to match ventilation with metabolic demand. Inhalation occurs when the forelimbs are not weight-bearing and are being protracted, and exhalation occurs during the support phase of the forelimbs, when the loading of the rib-cage (as well as the forward movement of the abdominal organs) helps drive air from the lungs. Therefore, as a horse gallops faster it breathes faster. As a horse becomes fatigued and stride frequency is reduced, it is noticeable that it lifts its centre of gravity further off the ground. This may occur to allow a lengthening of the inhalation phase in order to meet the oxygen deficit. The theoretical maximum respiratory rate would be 180 per minute, but at this rate the horse would not have any contact with the ground and would be flying. It takes the horse about twenty strides to establish the correct synchronisation between its gait and its breathing. The fact that breathing is not merely a passive flow of air into the lungs means that there is a price to be paid for getting the oxygen down into the alveoli. The work carried out in doing this by the respiratory muscles while the horse is at rest, is only a small fraction of the resting energy turnover. When the horse is working hard, however, the energy cost of breathing is relatively more 'expensive'.

The volume of air which a horse takes in at rest is something in the region of 100-150 litres per minute, requiring about 12-20 breaths.

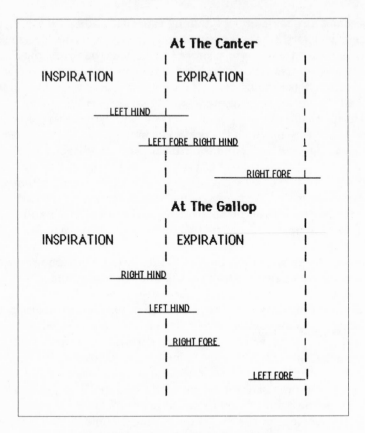

Fig 33 The timing of stride and respiration

However, with exercise, there is an increase in both respiratory rate and ventilation per minute so that the gallop ventilation may reach 1,600 litres per minute involving 140 breaths. The uptake of oxygen from the inspired air is greater during exercise than rest, probably reflecting the greater perfusion of the alveoli. In order to ensure that the maximum amount of air flows to the alveoli, the airways have to be dilated; this occurs owing to the release of adrenalin and nor-adrenalin. However, certain situations occur when the opposite happens, ie the airways are constricted. For example, in humans, the reasons that asthmatics become breathless is that the airways become constricted owing to an allergic reaction releasing histamine. As already discussed, a similar situation occurs in horses suffering from COPD. This is important because as ventilation increases so does the tidal volume, ie the volume of air taken in at one breath increases, as well as the speed of the air-flow along the airways. Therefore, as ventilation increases, the effects of any obstruction of air-flow becomes more prominent. Fitness does not appear to affect small airway obstruction such as COPD (contrary to what is sometimes claimed). Regular fast work may help mucus removal from down in the lungs, but the main obstructive effect of the bronchoconstriction will be unchanged.

In the normal galloping horse, all the air in the lungs is breathed out in half the time it takes for one stride. Horses which are suffering from the so-called 'loss of performance syndrome' after a respiratory infection, will not be able to get rid of all the air within this time (Fig 34). A horse with severe chronic obstructive pulmonary disease may take two or three strides to empty its lungs completely. Because of the natural link which exists between the horse's stride and its breathing, this markedly slows the horse's stride rate. So, the athletic horse with COPD will have reduced performance on two counts. First, it will not be achieving proper oxygenation of the blood in its lungs, depriving the muscles of sufficient oxygen to allow them to work as well as they might otherwise

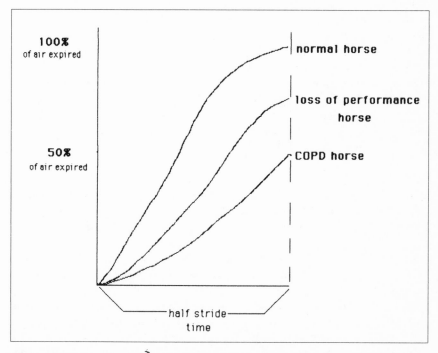

Fig 34 The percentage of the air in the horse's lung which can be expired during half a stride

do. Secondly, it will not be able to increase its stride rate as much as it might wish to do, and as it cannot significantly increase its stride length, then its speed will be restricted.

The physical act of breathing can be considered to have three stages:

1 Expansion of the thorax by the diaphragm, the intercostal muscles and other thoracic muscles.
2 The inspiration of atmospheric air and its mixing with the gases which have remained in the lungs after the horse has breathed out.
3 The diffusion of oxygen into the blood and of carbon dioxide in the reverse direction.

Anything which limits one or more of the above processes affects respiratory efficiency adversely. Expansion of the thorax may be affected by injury or disease, by pain, or by muscle weakness. The last point is probably rarely considered by horse owners, but it is self-evident that the powerful and rapid thoracic expansions necessary for a gallop require strong and fit respiratory muscles. While there is no direct evidence that proves that the diaghragm becomes stronger as a horse gets fitter, it is safe to assume that, like other muscles, it does so during a training regime. We have already seen that any condition which obstructs the flow of gas in any part of the lower respiratory system immediately affects respiratory efficiency. Virtually all inflammatory or allergic conditions have this effect because they cause narrowing or blockage of the airways, particularly the smaller ones which are so vulnerable to the slightest swelling of their pulmonary membranes. These membranes are sensitive to a great variety of damaging agents. There are few owners whose horses have never been exposed to infection or allergy at some stage of their lives.

Bleeders

Recent studies using fibre optic endoscopes have shown that following fast strenuous exercise up to 70 per cent of horses have spots of fresh blood along the trachea and lower airways. This has been called exercise-induced pulmonary haemorrhage (EIPH). If the haemorrhage is very marked, then blood may be seen at the nostrils, and referred to as epistaxis. For many years this blood was thought to be due to a nosebleed, although we now know that this is not the case. More recently, such horses have been said to have 'broken a blood-vessel', which is much nearer the mark. Although the occurrence of EIPH is variable, with blood not always being present in each individual horse after racing, horses where it is severe enough to cause blood at the nostrils, tend to suffer repeatedly from the problem. It would appear that it is fast work which produces the problem, because endurance horses do not show any blood in their lungs even at the end of very long and gruelling rides. Even with fast work there appears to be more to it than just the speed element. Working a horse on its own may not cause any blood to appear, whereas working it in 'competition' alongside another horse will do so even at the same or slower speeds.

There have been a variety of attempts to treat the condition, the most popular of which has been the use of frusemide, a diuretic which causes increased urine production. The theory was that the EIPH was due to congestion in the lungs, and the diuretic lessened this congestion by taking away the fluid. Whether this drug has any effect on reducing the severity of EIPH is controversial, with reports indicating no effect or a slight beneficial response. The actual cause of the haemorrhage is not known. It may be a perfectly normal response to severe exercise. On the other hand, it may be a response to viral infections or to COPD. At present, the best way of avoiding the problem is probably to keep the horse in as clean an environment as possible, both from the standpoint of infection and of dust, etc. It must be realised, however, that just because a horse does not visibly 'bleed' does not mean that it is not showing EIPH; it simply means that the blood has not come out of the nose. Endoscopic examination of the horse would probably still show blood in the lungs. As the proverb says, this is a case of 'What the eye does not see, the heart does not grieve over'.

Horsemen know that a training programme improves a horse's 'wind', by which they mean that its breathing after a gallop is not so laboured or noisy. Trainers might tell an owner that 'he could not blow a candle out after a gallop', a picturesque way of illustrating the point. The question is, what changes take place within the horse's whole respiratory system to bring about this effect of training? Although the most direct effect relates to the lung tissue itself, we have not yet found a way of measuring this. Nevertheless, it is probable that the patency of airways and the efficiency of the lung membranes are all greatly enhanced by training and correct nutrition. The indirect effects, on the other hand, have been measured and are well corroborated. Owing to the strengthening effect of training on the heart muscle and an increase in the haemoglobin content of the blood, the uptake of oxygen into the blood from the lungs is increased, allowing a matching to the increased oxidative capacity of the muscle. The end results of these effects of training is a reduction of the oxygen debt which the horse incurs during a gallop. A fit horse therefore recovers much faster after exercise than an unfit horse because it does not have to breathe in as much air in order to repay the oxygen debt. Whether this shows as a slower respiratory rate after exercise, or as a less marked increase in the thoracic movements, an observer notes an 'improvement in the wind'.

Causes of lost performance

Ever since the general public became aware of the existence of viruses as invisible particles which could cause respiratory diseases, such as the common cold, for which, unlike bacterial diseases, there was no cure, an increasing number of horse trainers have blamed poor performance on viruses. Some have gone so far as to refer to 'the virus' as if there was but one virus which caused all their problems. As a result, it may be that some of the other causes of poor performance, such as over-training, lack of proper work or even lack of ability, are now overlooked. When a large percentage of the horses in a yard appear to lose their form at the same time, it might well be that they are suffering from what has become called the 'poor performance syndrome'.

Among the symptoms commonly associated with this problem are:

1 Unexpected poor performance at fast speeds.
2 Excessive fatigue or respiratory distress after fast work.
3 Poor appetite.
4 Temperature varying from normal up to 105.8°F (41°C).
5 Staring coat.
6 Discharge from the nose and possibly the eyes.
7 Swelling of the lymph nodes around the jaw and larynx.
8 Coughing.
9 Small dry or moist, foul-smelling faeces.
10 Stiffness before or after exercise.

Most of these symptoms can be associated with a virus infection of the horse's upper respiratory tract. However, a variety of viruses might be involved; indeed, there may be a combination of infections causing the symptoms at any one time. Equine influenza virus, equine herpes virus 1 (rhinopneumonitis), rhinoviruses, and adenovirus may all be involved.

One of the reasons that viruses are often blamed for poor performance is that their diagnosis can be difficult, so it is a possibility which cannot easily be disproved. It is possible to isolate the virus itself, however. To do this swabs are taken from the horse's pharynx and inoculated onto tissue culture. Generally, this technique is most likely to be successful if carried out while the horse is running a high temperature, ie during the very early stages of the infection. In many cases, by the time the trainer has called in the veterinary surgeon, this stage is already over. A precise diagnosis may still be possible, however. If blood samples are taken as soon as possible after the development of any symptoms, and follow-up samples taken fourteen days later, these can be used to measure the amount of antibody present against the various viruses under suspicion. A high level of antibody against a virus in the initial sample does not mean that the virus is involved, because that antibody was made at least ten to fourteen days previously, as we have already discussed. A fourfold rise in the level of antibody present between the initial and follow-up samples does mean that an active infection has been at work. Such methods of diagnosis are, of necessity, time-consuming. As we discussed in the chapter on the cardiovascular system, it is not possible to make a diagnosis of respiratory virus infection purely on the basis of counting the blood cells present. They may provide clues, but not definite answers.

Equine herpes viruses complicate the problem even further because they can produce a situation known as latency. This means that all the horse's responses to the virus die down but the virus is still present somewhere in the body (as yet we do not know where). At a later stage this virus might be reactivated and multiply. It will then be shed out into the environment and infect other in-contact horses. It is thus possible to explain how an outbreak of coughing, etc can suddenly appear in a yard where there has been no known contact with the disease. Even if clinical symptoms are so slight that they are not spotted by the trainer, the very fact that a virus is actively present and multiplying is likely to affect performance. Indeed, it is possible that continued reactivation of the virus in different horses in a yard is responsible for the fact that the 'poor performance syndrome' can continue for many months.

Among the situations which are thought to stimulate reactivation of a latent virus are weaning, castration, breaking and transportation. In animals as a whole, reactivation can be triggered off by stress. There can be few things more stressful than a hard race. Is it coincidence that some horses take much longer than was expected to get over a hard race, or over a race which involved lengthy travel? At this stage we do not know. We do know, however, that giving a corticosteroid to a horse can reactivate a latent virus. This is important therapeutically, and may make one think twice about using corticosteroids in horses in training, etc. It is also significant because exercise is known to increase the levels of cortisol (the natural corticosteroid) in the blood, and this might be one of the reasons why the stress of racing, etc causes reactivation of the virus.

Vaccination against respiratory viruses
Influenza vaccines
All currently available vaccines against equine influenza contain whole virus which has been chemically inactivated. Such vaccines are there-

a

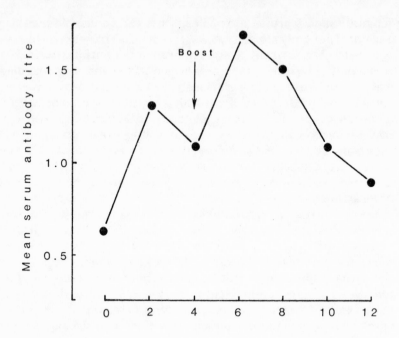

b

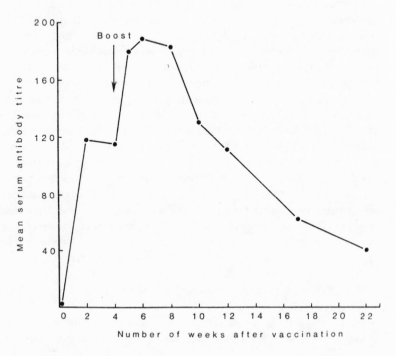

fore incapable of causing even a mild form of influenza. Although there has been a lot of concern and comment passed by trainers on detrimental side effects following influenza vaccination, this worry is not supported by the available evidence. From a survey carried out between 1981 and 1985 in Great Britain the reported reaction rate to influenza vaccine with or without tetanus was only 1 in 10,000. Of the reactions, almost 50 per cent were local. There are two subtypes of equine influenza both of which are included in the vaccines. Some vaccines contain adjuvants which enhance the immune response stimulated by the vaccine. Vaccination schedules recommended by the manufacturers should always be followed as a minimum requirement. These usually require a primary course of two doses given approximately four to eight weeks apart, followed by the first booster dose at six months, and thereafter at six to nine month intervals. In young animals immunity wanes rapidly, and additional doses may be advisable if the animal is likely to be put at risk of being infected, eg travelling abroad, visiting a show. In older animals (eight years) that have been regularly vaccinated, immunity persists for longer and annual booster doses may suffice. The immune status of an animal can be established by measuring serum antibody levels to ascertain whether re-vaccination is required.

Equid herpesvirus 1 (EHV–1) vaccines
There are two EHV–1 vaccines currently available in the United Kingdom. One vaccine is a live attenuated vaccine which is licensed for use against respiratory disease; the other is an inactivated vaccine which is licensed for the prevention of abortion. There are two subtypes of EHV–1: subtype 1 is the abortigenic form but is also capable of causing respiratory disease and paralysis; subtype 2 is the respiratory form and only occasionally has been associated with isolated abortions. Both vaccines contain the subtype 1 abortigenic virus only, and are therefore less likely to be as effective against the respiratory strain. Immunity provided by both vaccine is short-lived and the vaccination schedules recommended may be regarded as the minimum requirement to maintain a level of immunity. In young animals, a primary course of 2 x 2ml doses (three to four weeks apart Pneumabort-K[R], four to eight weeks apart Rhinomune[R]) followed by a six-month booster, is recommended, but those vaccines are sometimes administered as often as every three

Fig 35 The response of serum antibodies to vaccinations a) following dose of Pneumabort-K at 0 and 4 weeks, b) following Influenza Vaccine at 0 and 4 weeks. Note vastly differing serum titres against the two viruses is a result of different methods of measuring the titres. (Modified from Vet. Rec. (1984) Vol 114, 375-381 J. HYG. (CAMB). (1983) Vol 90, 371-384.)

months. When the inactivated vaccine is to be used in the prevention of abortion, pregnant mares are vaccinated in the fifth, seventh and ninth months of gestation. However, it is advisable that mares are also vaccinated prior to the fifth month as some abortions occur in the fourth month of gestation.

The inactivated vaccine contains an oil-based adjuvant which may on occasions produce a local reaction at the site of injection. The live vaccine is administered intramuscularly, and it is claimed that there is no subsequent virus shedding from the respiratory tract. There have been reports, however, that virus indistinguishable from vaccine virus has been isolated from the occasional aborted foetus.

7 · Thermoregulation

All the activities of the millions of cells in the horse's body are dependent on the production and utilisation of energy. This energy may be in the form of chemical, mechanical, or heat energy. In many instances, the amount of heat produced is greater than that needed by the horse for its normal body functions. The horse must lose this excess heat in order to maintain a relatively constant body temperature because extremes of body temperature can be dangerous.

Heat production inside the horse's body
Most of the horse's body heat is produced during the breakdown of feedstuffs and the 'burning' of oxygen. In the resting horse, the amount of heat produced by the muscles is relatively small because they are inactive. During exercise, however, there is an increased production of heat as the muscles start to work. In fact, there is a large increase in heat production because the conversion of chemical energy (from substances such as glycogen and glucose) into mechanical energy is relatively inefficient. About 75 per cent of the energy produced will be in the form of heat. The total amount of heat produced will depend both on which muscles are involved in that particular activity (the bigger the muscle involved, the more heat that will be produced) and the number of muscle contractions which occur in that time. Even at gentle exercise, heat production can increase by between ten and twenty times that produced at rest. During sprinting, it can rise to between forty and fifty times the resting amount.

When the horse is working so hard that it requires more energy than it can obtain from the oxygen it breathes in, it will also have to break down carbohydrates to lactate in order to produce more energy. It will therefore produce even more heat from this chemical reaction. What many people do not realise is that in this case extra heat will continue to be produced even after the horse stops exercising because the lactate has to be broken down during the recovery period and this produces more heat. The more strenuous the exercise, the more lactate that will have to be removed, and the longer time it will take before the horse returns to just resting heat-production levels. Needless to say, if the horse is also absorbing heat from high environmental temperature or high solar radiation, the build-up of heat during exercise will be exacerbated.

The horse must obviously have some mechanism for losing all this heat because under normal conditions its body temperature remains at around 101°F (38°C) when measured with a rectal thermometer. This rectal temperature is considered to approximate closely to the true or central core body temperature. There is a gradual lowering of this central core temperature from the centre of the horse out towards the skin. When the horse is resting, the temperature of its muscles at 98.2°F (36.8°C) is slightly below its rectal temperature because at this time the blood supply to the muscles is relatively low. The normal body temperature is quite close to the temperature which can threaten life if it is maintained for any length of time. In the horse this critical temperature is considered to be above 105.8°F (41°C).

As the horse's body temperature increases, so do the rates of the various body processes which produce heat. It can become rather like a vicious circle: the higher the horse's body temperature, the more heat that will be generated, and so there is a further increase in temperature. At temperatures above 111.2°F (44°C) actual breakdown of tissue proteins occurs.

When a horse works sufficiently to raise its heart rate to approximately 150 beats per minute (which is about 50 per cent of maximum oxygen uptake), every three minutes of exercise will raise its body temperature by 1.8°F (1°C). So, after about ten minutes the horse's body temperature would be within the critical level. If the horse worked harder, the critical level would obviously be reached even sooner. Fortunately, these increases in body temperature do not usually occur because the horse has developed a number of mechanisms whereby it can quickly dissipate this extra heat into the environment. The general term for these mechanisms is thermoregulation. Although few studies have been carried out in the horse, it is apparent that the horse has a very effective thermoregulatory system and is only rarely troubled by hyperthermia caused by either environmental conditions, exercise or a combination of both.

How the horse loses heat

With so much heat being produced in the athletic horse, it must obviously have some means of losing this heat, especially from the muscles during exercise. This is helped by an efficient circulatory system. The blood passing through the tissues is able to 'take up' the heat from the cells and then transport it to areas from which it can be lost to the air.

Blood is able to carry a great deal of heat with only a moderate increase in its own temperature.

In the horse, as in man and a few other species, the major loss of heat to the environment is via the skin. Only a minor portion of the heat is lost from the respiratory system during breathing because the expired air becomes saturated with water vapour. This dominant role of the skin in cooling the horse is the reason why the blood-vessels become so prominent over the skin during exercise. As the veins returning blood from the extremities are so near the surface, effective heat exchange can occur. The increased blood flow to the horse's skin during and after exercise raises the skin's temperature and, as long as the environmental temperature is below that of the skin, heat loss can occur down a thermal gradient.

Table 8   Heat loss from the skin

1	Conduction	Of minor importance.
2	Radiation	Of minor importance.
3	Convection	Related to the air velocity and the temperature gradient
4	Evaporation	The most important source of heat loss.

Of the various mechanisms of heat loss, conduction is generally of minor importance (Table 8). Convection is related to air velocity, so the greater the wind (or the greater the horse's speed) the greater the heat loss possible. Radiation is dependent on a temperature gradient between the skin and the environment. If, on the other hand, the environmental temperature is higher than the skin temperature, absorption of heat will occur and this will increase the heat load to be lost by other mechanisms. This situation occurs quite often in tropical countries. The final major mechanism for heat loss, and one which can operate even when the environmental temperature is higher than that of the skin, is evaporation, ie the vaporisation of water from the surfaces of the skin and the respiratory system.

The advantages and disadvantages of sweating

In the resting horse, where excess heat production is minimal, most of the heat loss is via convection, radiation and evaporation from the respiratory system during normal breathing. However, these mechanisms cannot cope with the large increases in heat production which occur during exercise, and the evaporation of sweat then becomes the major means of heat loss. The effectiveness of this particular mechanism lies in the fact that for every litre of water (weighing 2.2lb (1kg)) that is vaporised, approximately 580 kilocalories (2.4 megajoules) of heat are removed from the body. In other words, the evaporation of 1 litre of water from the body will remove the heat produced by 'burning' 120 litres of oxygen. With completely effective sweating, a horse working at 50 per cent of maximum oxygen uptake will take an hour to lose 16 litres of sweat. A racehorse which is only racing for about two minutes will only lose 1–1½ litres so water loss is minimal during short bursts of maximal exercise and it should not pose any problems. Obviously, these figures will be lower in cooler and windy conditions where convection and radiation can also contribute to the losses. In one 50 mile (80km) endurance ride under cool conditions, carried out at a speed of 5mph (8kmph), a total loss of about 37 litres occurred. This represents a loss of 7½ litres of sweat every hour of the ride.

Whether the maximum possible amount of heat loss from sweating does occur is dependent on the external environment. In a hot, dry atmosphere, evaporative cooling is highly efficient. In high humidity, however, sweating may be inefficient because up to two-thirds of the sweat will run off the skin before it can be evaporated. Any prolonged exercise under these conditions can be a health threat to the horse. It is important to realise that sweat dropping freely from the horse indicates an effective sweating mechanism but a very inefficient cooling mechanism, the two things are not synonymous. In other words, a horse which is only slightly wet with sweat may be losing more heat by rapid evaporation of its sweat than one which literally has sweat pouring off it. Incidentally, coat thickness appears to influence sweating efficiency. A thick coat in the winter is not only a better insulation against the cold weather, it also allows less heat loss from sweating.

As air temperature, wind velocity and relative humidity all influence the various mechanisms by which the horse loses heat, the effectiveness of its heat loss and the subsequent risk of it overheating will vary under different climatic conditions. From time to time, equine competitions are held in conditions which may give rise to serious problems on this score, and there is then a great demand for some sort of guideline which will safeguard the welfare of the horses being asked to take part. The more important the competition, the more critical the public will be if a wrong decision is taken as to whether or not the competition should take place. To try to estimate the effectiveness of heat dissipation and the risks to the health of competitors, both human and equine, taking part in athletic activities, a number of systems have been suggested which will evaluate the factors influencing heat loss.

When does the climate make it unsafe to compete?
In man, one system used is that in which a dry-bulb temperature (db),

wet-bulb temperature (wb) which represents the humidity, and the black-globe temperature (bg) which represents the radiation, are all measured. The following formula is then used to calculate the Wet-Bulb Globe Temperature (WBGT).

WBGT °F = $(0.7 \times wb) + (0.2 \times bg) + (0.1 \times db)$

From experience with this scale, the following precautions have been suggested in human sports activities:

WBGT	Precautions
80–85°F	Caution! Frequent water breaks
85–88°F	Limited activity for trained people
88°F+	No activity allowed

For example, if the wet-bulb temperature is 75°F, the black-globe temperature is 110°F and the dry-bulb temperature is 85°F then

WBGT = $(75 \times 0.7) + (110 \times 0.2) + (85 \times 0.1) = 83°F$

A more simple system has been proposed to determine an 'effective temperature' to prevent excess heat build up in equine endurance rides. This is the sum of the ambient temperature in degrees Fahrenheit and the relative humidity. When the sum is less than 130, heat loss should not be a problem. Higher than 150, especially if the relative humidity contributes more than half the sum, then evaporative cooling is severely compromised and so caution is needed. A figure over 180 means that normal cooling will be almost completely ineffectual, and so exercise should only continue for very brief periods. It would appear reasonable, therefore, to suggest that racing or any other sort of equine competition should not take place at all if the value is over 180. Between 150 and 180 the competitors should always be warned that caution is necessary, and they should be allowed to withdraw without penalty if they wish to do so.

Under most climatic conditions the regulatory mechanisms which we have described are able to provide sufficient thermoregulatory control of the horse's body. However, where heat production is very great over a period of time, the role of the respiratory system may become more important. In such conditions, the horse may start to pant. This is actually a form of rapid, shallow breathing in which the air is moved rapidly in and out of the upper respiratory tract. In a hot, humid environment respiratory rates of over 200 per minute have been recorded. One way in which this use of the respiratory system to cool down the horse's body shows during competitions is when endurance rides are held in hot, humid conditions. In such cases the respiratory rate exceeds the heart rate during the post-ride recovery period. In cooler climates, this inversion of the normal relationship between pulse rate and respiratory rate is not generally seen.

Despite all these mechanisms to enable the horse to lose heat, usually a small rise in central core temperature is seen in addition to the expected rise in muscle temperature. Therefore, a small rise in rectal temperature after a competition should not be viewed with alarm as long as it is below the critical level of 105.8°F (41°C). The raised body temperature is a form of heat storage, with the heat being gradually lost once the exercise is over. This ability to store some of the heat produced was developed in a number of large mammals and it has been suggested that, especially in desert animals, eg the camel, it is a useful adaptation because it reduces water loss. A small rise in muscle temperature is also not a bad thing for the athletic horse. It leads to a better muscle contraction, hence the value of a pre-competition warm up.

Where does sweat come from and what does it contain?

As has already been mentioned, the major method of heat loss in the horse is by evaporation of water from the skin in the form of sweat. This sweat is formed in sweat glands down in the depths of the skin, next to the hair follicles. There are sweat glands all over the body, although there are higher concentrations of them in areas such as the horse's neck. Whether differences in sweating ability between different horses may be related to the horses possessing different numbers of sweat glands is not known. The glands start secreting sweat when they are told to do so by hormones in the bloodstream. There are two hormones involved: adrenalin, which is released during exercise, and nor-adrenalin, which is released by nerves. It is because of these adrenalins that horses sweat when they become excited. A higher sensitivity to adrenalin probably explains why warm-blooded horses such as Thoroughbreds sweat more readily than cold-blooded horses.

Table 9 Approximate concentration of major electrolytes in 1 litre of sweat

	Sodium		*Potassium*		*Chloride*	
	mmol/l	g/l	mmol/l	g/l	mmol/l	g/l
Plasma	140	3.2	4.0	.16	100	3.5
Horse sweat	160	3.7	35	1.4	175	6.2
Human sweat	35	0.75	4.5	.18	35	1.2

Note: 1oz = 28.3g

As is well known, sweat is not just pure water. Dissolved within it are other substances such as electrolytes. The major electrolytes, or salts, present are sodium, potassium and chloride. In contrast to the sweat formed by human beings, large amounts of the above-mentioned electrolytes (as well as calcium and magnesium) are lost from the horse during sweating (Table 9). This means that, at a similar rate of sweating to a man, a horse will lose about three times as much sodium chloride and five to ten times as much potassium as the man.

Recently, there has been renewed interest in the large amounts of proteins which have been found in horse sweat. This is also in contrast to the situation in man where there are only negligible amounts of proteins. Although this high-protein content has been known since the turn of the century, and has been suggested as representing potentially an important protein loss to the horse, new research has now shown the nature and function of these proteins. First, it has been found that high-protein concentrations are only seen during the early stages of sweating, and the levels then gradually decrease. So, the protein loss is not as great as originally thought when it was assumed that a constantly high level of protein was being lost. Secondly, the proteins found in the sweat glands are of a special type and their nature suggests that they have detergent-like properties. This means that they aid in the dispersion of the sweat droplets into a thin film along the hairs, and this helps evaporation. We are able, therefore, to explain some observations known to all horsemen, ie that sweat readily lathers, and also that as the horse becomes fitter the sweat becomes more watery. In horses exercised frequently (and so presumably becoming fitter), the protein content of the sweat decreases because the time required for its replacement cannot keep pace with the rate of its secretion in the sweat. A very high-power picture of a sweat gland and the vesicles containing the protein is shown in Plate 20. With sweating continuing over many hours, there may be a decrease in the rate of sweat production, and this can lead to a loss in thermoregulatory capacity. This occurs as the cells within the sweat gland become fatigued.

Dry coat
Anhydrosis (dry coat) is the term used to describe the condition in which horses develop either partial or complete inability to sweat in the usual way. This condition was first recognised by the British when horses were shipped from Britain to their tropical colonies, and then developed the problem. Today, it is seen in numerous tropical countries, eg Hong Kong, Malaysia, India, northern Australia and the gulf states of the USA. It was originally thought that anhydrosis only occurred when horses were brought from a cool to a hot, humid climate, but it can also be seen in horses which have lived all their lives in such climates. It appears to be more common in Thoroughbreds or part-Thoroughbreds

than in cold-blooded breeds. Generally both high temperatures and high humidity are required for the condition to develop although it is seen in places where only extremely high temperatures occur, eg Arizona. Obviously, not all horses develop the disorder, but its incidence is high enough to warrant concern because the horses may be at risk if given even mild exercise. In Hong Kong an incidence of about 3 per cent is seen in horses imported from Britain, Australia and New Zealand for racing. These then have to be withdrawn from racing. Recently, a report from Florida suggested that up to 20 per cent of horses in the Miami area are affected during the summer months, which makes anhydrosis of great concern financially as well as from the welfare point of view. It is unknown whether there is any genetic predisposition to the disorder, nor is it known whether any test can be developed to predict if a horse is predisposed to it. Although development has generally been associated with exercise, it has also been reported in resting stabled horses and brood mares.

The signs associated with anhydrosis are panting and a dry coat. Occasionally, the horse loses its appetite and starts to lose weight. The coat becomes poor in condition and there may be alopecia, or loss of hair. Anhydrosis can start suddenly or gradually, and may or may not be associated with visible sweating beforehand.

Why horses become either partially or completely anhydrotic is at present unknown. However, recent research has indicated that it is probably due to many of the sweat glands losing their ability to function properly because the cells producing the sweat have become exhausted and their internal structure changed. This suggests that an abnormal period of prolonged sweating must have occurred, leading to temporary damage to the glands. Although a number of treatments have been tried on such horses, they have generally been unsuccessful and the only effective means of treatment is to remove the horse to a more temperate climate. In hot, humid environments the condition may be avoided by stabling horses in air-conditioned stables. In affected animals the sweat glands recover during the cooler months of the year, but the condition reoccurs the following summer.

The importance of water to the athletic horse

In the horse, as in any other animal, the total amount of water in the body is around 60 per cent of the body-weight. In other words, a 1,100lb (500kg) horse will contain about 65½gal (300 litres) of water. Of this water, two-thirds are found within the body's cells (ie it is extracellular), while the other third is found in the plasma, or fluid phase of the blood, between cells and in the gastro-intestinal tract (ie it is extracellular). It is often forgotten that about 6–10 per cent of the horse's weight is intestinal fluid, and part of this fluid can act as a reservoir for the exercising horse. The horse is able to maintain its water content fairly precisely by adjusting the amount of fluid it takes in. This is done via internal sensors which react to changes in the circulating blood volume and to increases in the amounts of sugar, proteins and electrolytes within the circulation. The sensors can then send messages to the brain to activate the thirst centre and thus to stimulate drinking.

Although a great deal has been written on the watering of horses, much of the advice given has had little foundation in facts and is often contradictory. Much of the information, for example, has been handed down and perpetuated from articles written in the last century, at a time when, for various reasons, water was rationed and only given at fixed times. Unfortunately, no easy recipe can be given for the amount of water a horse requires as this will vary according to age, size of horse, environmental temperature and relative humidity, amount of work the horse is engaged in and the type of food it is receiving. Both dry, bulky feeds and high-protein feeds will increase the amount of water required. Obviously, factors such as whether its work causes sweating will also increase a horse's water requirements. The daily water requirement will vary between 4 and 17gal (20 and 80 litres). In order to satisfy such a varying demand, it is best if an unlimited supply of water is available. Although this is best provided by one of the automatic watering systems, if one of these is not available (as will often be the case), water should be provided in clean buckets or troughs which are frequently emptied and replaced with fresh, clean water. Either way, it is important that horses should be allowed to drink when they wish, and this overcomes questions about the desirability of watering before competitions or other work. As far as quality and temperature of the water are concerned, it appears that neither the degree of hardness nor the temperature of the water is of any practical importance. There appears little evidence that cold water will lead to colic; in the horse that has been working, cold water in the digestive tract will help in the cooling of the central core temperature which, as we discussed earlier, might have been raised by the exercise.

From research carried out in ponies, we know that it is extremely important that water is available both before, during and after feeding because in the wild state horses are periprandial drinkers. This rather grand term means that they usually drink around the time of feeding. The advice often given not to water horses around feeding time is obviously contrary to this natural habit. During exercise of prolonged duration, especially where either the speed of the horse or the environmental conditions cause sweating, water should be made available at regular intervals. In people competing in marathon running, it has now been found that drinks should be made available soon after the start as well as during the later stages, as was previously the custom. It is also considered that fluid is usually only necessary for human athletes during competitions lasting more than one hour.

It would seem sensible to encourage horses to drink during all rest stages of competitions requiring marked physical effort. Research in the USA has shown that horses drink copiously during endurance rides held under hot, still conditions, with no apparent ill effects. Despite this, they will still finish with a slight degree of dehydration. As long as they are allowed free access to water during the recovery period, most of this water loss will be rapidly replaced. As some horses will not drink automatically during prolonged exercise (whether naturally or due to prior conditioning from human training we do not know), it may be necessary to train them to develop a habit of drinking whenever given the opportunity to do so.

When water loss does occur, it is mainly from the extracellular stores, especially from the interstitial compartment, the water which lies between the various tissues of the horse's body. The loss from this compartment is why one of the most easily applied tests for determining the degree of dehydration is so useful. The pinch test, as it is called, measures the speed of recoil of a pinched piece of skin. It is best applied over the neck or shoulder region. In a normal hydrated horse, recoil is almost immediate. However, with increasing dehydration this recoil becomes delayed because the removal of water from between the tissues decreases their elasticity. Changes in this skin elasticity become obvious when the horse has lost between 3 and 5 per cent of its body-weight in water loss. Although the effects of moderate dehydration, ie up to a 5 per cent loss in body-weight, have not been studied in horses, in man it has been shown that there is an adverse effect on work performance with fluid losses equivalent to between 2 and 4 per cent of body-weight.

Electrolytes and their relationship to dehydration
As we have already mentioned, there are other substances lost in sweat as well as water. Of these, the most important from the point of view of the horse's continued well-being is the loss of electrolytes. Electrolytes,

Plate 14 The application of faradic stimulation for muscle diagnosis and treatment

Plate 15 A cold laser machine

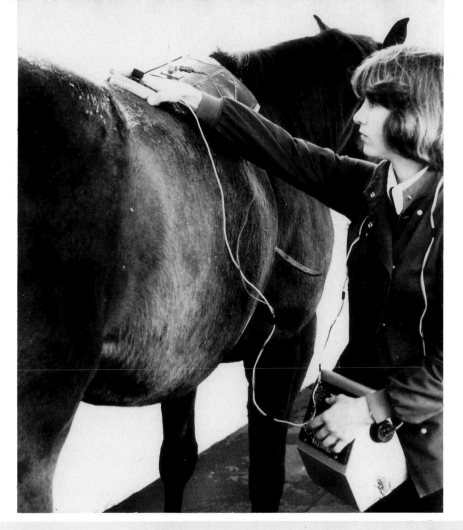

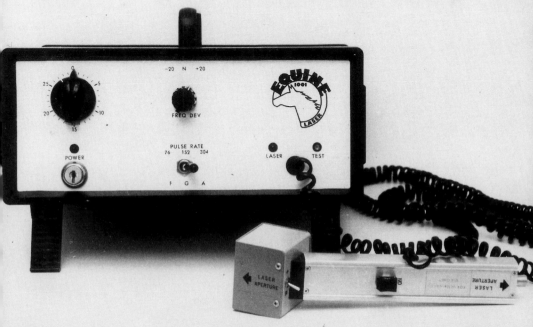

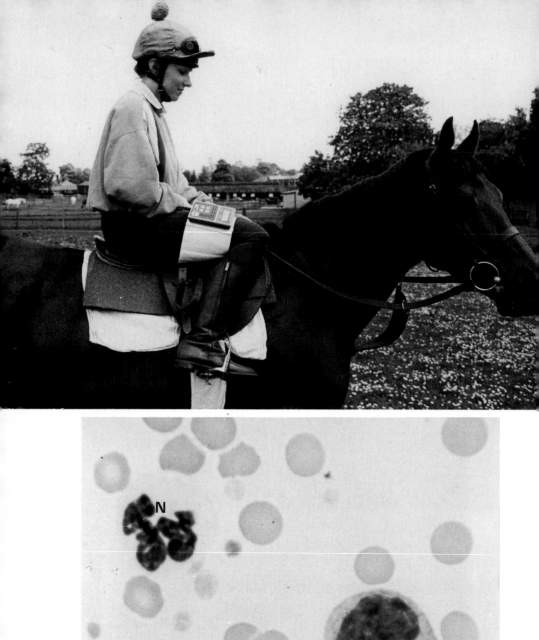

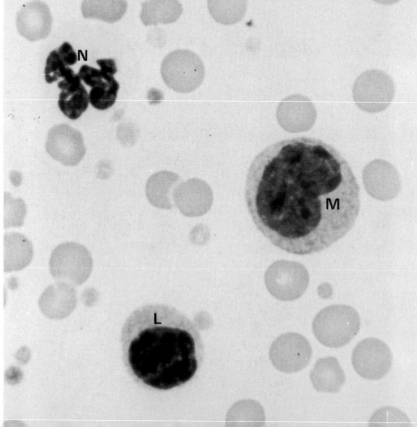

which are also referred to as salts or minerals, are elements which carry either a positive or negative electrical charge. They are found in various combinations. Common salt, for example, is a combination of equal amounts of sodium and chloride. The main electrolytes found in the horse's body are sodium, potassium, calcium, magnesium, chloride and phophorus (in the form of phosphate). Others which are required in smaller amounts are referred to as trace elements, and these include iron, copper, zinc, cobalt, selenium, sulphur and iodine. All of them have important roles within the body in ensuring that it functions normally. Many are important in several different ways. Calcium, for instance, is important in controlling many metabolic pathways, in the contraction of muscle fibres and as an important constituent of bone, so a calcium deficiency can lead to various disorders. The major electrolytes are potassium, sodium and chloride. Their proportions in the different compartments of the horse's body are shown in Table 10. As can be seen, potassium is mainly found within the actual cells, while sodium and chloride are found in the extra-cellular compartment. This is thought to be the result of the situation when all forms of life were restricted to the sea, and the cells were bathed by sea water.

Table 10   Normal amounts of water and major electrolytes in the body of a 500kg horse

	Water (litres)	Sodium (moles)	Potassium (moles)	Chloride (moles)
Intracellular fluid	183	2	27.5	1
Interstitial fluid	93	13	0.3	10.6
Blood plasma	24	3.3	0.1	2.3
Total amount	300	18	28	14

(A mole is a measurement of the number of molecules and one ounce (28.3g) of common salt (ie NaCl) contains about half a mole of both sodium and chloride)

Under normal conditions, the adult horse or pony being fed a ration adequate to satisfy its energy needs should be receiving sufficient amounts of the required electrolytes, and should not therefore develop

Plate 16 A cardiotachometer (Equistat – EQB, USA). This is one of the commercially available meters. The electrodes are placed under the saddle at the wither and on the bottom of chest under the girth strap. The electrodes are connected to the meter which can be attached to the rider's thigh or forearm. Heart rates are continually monitored via a digital readout. A stopwatch facility also allows timing of particular intervals in an exercise period

Plate 17 There are different types of white blood cells. The major ones are neutrophils (N), lymphocytes (L) and monocytes (M)

any disorders associated with electrolyte disturbances. There are a few exceptions to this. Horses grazing pastures where the soil is deficient in selenium or iodine, for example, may well develop problems. Problems can also arise from diets containing inappropriated calcium/phosphate ratios, eg when excessive bran is fed. Normally, however, the diet contains an excess of these electrolytes and by a number of complex regulatory mechanisms involving the release of several hormones, the horse is able to maintain its electrolyte concentrations within a narrow range. Any excess electrolytes are excreted via the kidneys into the urine. It is important, therefore, to realise that because of these regulatory mechanisms the horse is not able to store any of these electrolytes, and so anything which will lead to shortages will rapidly become obvious. Another fact which follows from this is that there is no point in trying to feed a horse with electrolytes during the evening or morning before a competition.

The two most common causes of electrolyte deficiencies are those brought about by diarrhoea and those resulting from profuse sweating. In the athletic horse, the individuals most likely to be affected by electrolyte deficiencies are not those in strenuous exercise of a short duration, such as racehorses or showjumpers, but those in longer events, particularly endurance rides, where the sweat loss is much greater. However, as has been mentioned already, the losses will also always be greater in hot environments. It is not only during the competitions that these losses occur, but also during training programmes which require the horse to exercise for several hours each day. As a general rule, a horse which is sweating moderately heavily will be losing about 8¾pt (5 litres) of sweat per hour. Each litre of this sweat contains 7.5–10.5g sodium chloride and 1.5–3.5g potassium chloride. In a 50 mile (80km) ride held in a cool climate, Thoroughbreds were found to lose 8gal (3 litres) of sweat over a five-hour period. This corresponds to a loss of about ¾lb (350g) of salt, which is equivalent to between one-third and one-half of their total body sodium chloride content. Horses exercising at a fast pace in hot, dry climates will have sweat losses two or three times this amount.

From the above figures, it is evident that in prolonged exercise, as well as ensuring frequent access to water, electrolytes should also be given. It will not be possible to replace immediately all the salt which has been lost, as water with the same salt concentration as sweat would be too salty for the horse to drink. However, with training, it is possible to get horses to accept water which contains a degree of salt. If the horse will not take the salted water, it is still preferable in the short term to have it at least drink plain water rather than no water at all. At the end of the competition, salts should be added to the feed as well as to the drinking water.

Although in prolonged exercise immediate electrolyte replacement is important, for shorter periods of moderate exercise, ie one to two hours, it is not so important. However, as shown in Table 11, it is unlikely that the normal diet will provide sufficient sodium and possibly potassium to replace the losses, and so electrolytes should be added to either the water or the feed. Numerous supplements are available, but unfortunately few of these contain the correct proportions of sodium to potassium. A preparation should be used which contains four times as much sodium as potassium. When moderate sweating occurs, it may only be necessary to supplement with sodium, and by far the cheapest form of doing this is by using common table salt. One tablespoon of table salt contains approximately 17g of sodium chloride. Many electrolyte supplements also contain calcium and magnesium, and these may be helpful in replacing losses of these electrolytes. Another cheap alternative to using a commercial electrolyte supplement is to provide the horse with free access to a salt-lick or rock salt. However, if the horse is disinclined to use these licks, supplementation in the feed or water must be used. In some electrolyte preparations glucose, dextrose or citrate are added. These are included not as sources of energy but to increase the absorption of the electrolytes. For horses competing in prolonged endurance events, you should not use preparations containing bicarbonate.

Table 11 Sodium and potassium balance in the exercising horse

	Sodium (g)	Potassium (g)
Amount in feed/day (hard feed plus hay)	36	95
Daily requirements	14	60
Excess intake per day	22	35
Loss per hour of sweating	27	15
Situation after 1hr of sweating	−5	20
Situation after 3hr of sweating	−59	−10

Synchronous diaphragmatic flutter (the thumps) is a condition most frequently seen in endurance horses competing in hot climates. It is also occasionally seen in the USA in racehorses following the use of frusemide (Lasix) as a pre-race medication to try and prevent epistaxis or bleeding from the nose. It is a term used to describe a condition in which the diaphragm contracts in rhythm with the heart beat. It is seen as a twitch or spasm in the flank which is not related to the normal respiratory movements but which can become sufficiently violent to produce an audible thumping sound. It is often seen during the cooling off period after endurance rides. In itself it is not serious, but it is indicative of a significant electrolyte imbalance. For this reason the appearance of the condition will result in the veterinary surgeon removing the horse from the competition. The exact cause of the condition is unknown, but it can be treated by the injection of electrolyte solutions containing calcium. It may be prevented by the supply of electrolytes to the horse during the ride.

Heat stroke
Heat stroke, or hyperthermia, can develop rapidly in horses that have become anhydrotic. It can even occur in resting horses which are confined to hot, poorly ventilated stables. However, it is most likely to be seen in hot and humid conditions when thermo-regulation cannot keep pace with the heat produced in poorly conditioned and over-extended horses during exercise. It can occur either during heavy exercise over short periods, eg when the cross-country stages in eventing take place in very hot, humid climates, or in the later stages of an endurance ride when a horse has become markedly dehydrated owing to insufficient consumption of water. Dehydration results mainly from a loss of fluid from the extracellular fluid compartments, so in addition to the loss from the interstitial spaces which results in the loss of skin elasticity, marked losses occur from the vascular compartment. This means that the total circulating blood volume is reduced. Under these circumstances the blood supply to the muscles has to be maintained in order to continue the effort required, but there is reduced blood flow to the skin. As a result, there is less transfer of heat from the skin and a consequent build-up of heat within the horse's body to above the critical temperature. This maintenance of the blood flow to the muscles as an immediate life-saving mechanism in fleeing from danger means that it is up to the rider to regulate the horse's speed in hot, humid conditions because the horse's performance will not markedly decrease until an over-heated state is reached. The rider must reduce speed in unfavourable climates in order to avoid the risks of dehydration and, in the worst cases, heat stroke.

The clinical signs of heat stroke are depression, weakness, and a refusal to go on. Pulse and respiratory rates are markedly increased, and rectal temperatures may reach as high as 106–110°F (41.5–43°C). The skin feels hot and dry, and sweating is inadequate. In severe cases, the horse may start to sway and convulse before going into a coma and dying.

If the signs of heat stroke are seen, a veterinary surgeon should be called immediately, but as urgent treatment is needed, initial steps can be taken by the horse owner to lower rapidly the body temperature. The horse should be moved into the shade in a well-ventilated area, preferably in a breeze. Fans can be used if available to ensure a rapid flow of air over the horse's body. The horse should then be hosed or, if a hose is not available, its coat should be continually soaked with buckets of cool or cold water. If ice is available, it should be placed over the large veins which show up under the skin of the head, neck and legs. Ice-water enemas and cold-water drenches may also be used in an emergency to try to reduce the body temperature. It is *vital* that this temperature is reduced to normal levels as quickly as possible. A veterinary surgeon will give intravenous fluid therapy in order to restore an effective circulating blood volume. He will also administer other drugs as appropriate.

In many cases, heat stroke can be avoided by care from the rider. A horse should be well trained, and if the environmental conditions are unfavourable, speed should be considerably reduced to prevent heat build-up within the body. Even when heat stroke is not likely to occur, there is considerable controversy over what is the best and safest way to lower body temperature during and immediately following competitions. The hosing and ice-packs which have already been mentioned are universally used, but there is controversy over whether cold water should be applied to the major muscle masses. One school of thought is that this may lead to muscle cramp and tying-up, and should therefore be avoided. However, others believe that cold water has no detrimental effect, and this is supported by the fact that some endurance riders almost submerge their horses in rivers and streams when possible during the rides. If the water was too cold it may be self-defeating because it could lead to partial constriction, or closing, of the smaller blood-vessels and actually slow down heat transfer. Recently, a study of people suffering from heat stroke on a pilgrimage to Mecca found that evaporative cooling can be best achieved by spraying patients with water at 59°F (15°C) and blowing warm air at 86–95°F (30–35°C) over them. In the field, then, a garden spray could be used to spray continuously cool water over the horse's entire body and a fan could be used to create air movement and so allow evaporation in an obviously hot environment.

Can the horse adapt to hot climates?
Unfortunately, no research has been carried out into the ability of horses to adapt to hot environments, and into how long this may take. All that can be done is to call on the experiences and evidence from man, another species where sweating is the major thermoregulatory mechanism. It is well known that following several days of exposure to a hot climate, temperature tolerance is increased and less discomfort is

felt. This acclimatisation to heat is seen as a lower body temperature, lower pulse rate and readier sweating. It is the latter which is thought to be the main mechanism of acclimatisation as more effective sweating results in quicker heat loss with a lower skin temperature. Because of a greater sweating efficiency, less blood has to be diverted to the skin, and so the important blood flow to the muscles can be maintained. This then results in an increased work capacity for acclimatised animals compared with those that have not adapted.

Just as in man, it is likely that different horses have differing capacities to tolerate heat and that they also acclimatise at different rates. In man most of the acclimatisation occurs within four to seven days of heat exposure, and it is complete after about two weeks. It has been found that, during this acclimatisation, the sweating rate can increase by 100 per cent. From the discussion on anhydrosis, it is obvious that certain horses cannot acclimatise, and for some unknown reason these increased demands for sweating lead to fatigue. Heat acclimatisation is a subject which warrants further investigation in the horse. We need to know, for instance, how to select those horses most likely to adapt when introduced into hot climates. The period of acclimatisation is the reason why, even in temperate countries, medical problems can arise when competitions are held in a sudden hot spell after a cold winter. In this case the adaptations normally seen with a gradual rise in temperature have not occurred. It is likely that both thermoregulation and acclimatisation can be helped by clipping the coat as this aids efficient sweating. It has also been shown in man that a well-trained individual is better able to adjust to the heat than one who is unfit.

8 · Training for Performance

Now that we have described how the various parts of the body function during exercise, we can consider how this knowledge can help us to devise suitable training programmes for the different athletic activities. In the case of racing, it is the aim of trainers to realise a horse's full potential. Horses involved in leisure activities, on the other hand, may only require a limited degree of fitness because they will not often be performing at their maximum capability. The aim of training is obviously to increase a horse's fitness so that it can compete more successfully, and with less risk of injury, against horses of equal ability. It has been suggested that fatigue is the major cause of tendon breakdowns in racehorses, and it is certainly the main reason why horses fall at the last few fences of a steeplechase race. Training is very much involved in delaying the onset of fatigue during performance.

Recently, it has become fashionable to put forward the theory that progress in training methods for equine athletes has lagged behind developments for human athletes. It has been claimed, probably quite correctly, that the continued advancements in human athletic performance, as shown by the frequent setting of new world records, is largely due to a more scientific approach to training. Of course, this is not the entire story. Other factors, such as improved track surfaces and equipment, more professionalism (or sham amateurism) and the selection of athletes from an ever-widening population, all contribute to this improvement. When race records for Thoroughbreds and Standardbreds on both sides of the Atlantic are considered, however, only minimal improvements can be seen over the past fifty years. Where improvement has occurred, it has generally been in Standardbred racing, where there have been advances in track and cart (sulky) design and where the trainers have been ready to introduce new training methods. The least improvement has been seen in Thoroughbred circles, where trainers have retained traditional training methods. The present generation of Thoroughbred trainers, however, is becoming more and more receptive to new ideas.

Whether more scientifically based training methods will actually lead to marked improvements in race times has to be questioned on a number of grounds. Although selective breeding in horses has led to the evolution of animals for a specific task, eg the Thoroughbred and Standardbred, it may be that we have now achieved the optimum genetic state in this respect. In that case, further improvements will only be small compared with man where athletes are drawn from a very varied population. There are also psychological factors to consider. Much of the improvement in human athletics has come about because individuals are prepared to train at very high levels which result in pain and distress. Because of the financial and other incentives for success, the human athlete is willing to tolerate such possible abuse of his body. Fortunately, or unfortunately, depending on your point of view, one cannot expect the horse to be willing to be pushed to such an extent as these incentives are meaningless to it. For example, a colt cannot be told that he will have a stud career rather than possibly ending up as dog meat if he performs outstandingly. If a horse is pushed too hard not only are the risks of breakdown substantially increased, but also the experience of pain, associated either with the build-up of lactic acid during fatigue or with minor injuries, may sour it from racing altogether. So, horses often cannot be trained as hard as man.

It should be pointed out that the aim of this chapter is not to describe specific training programmes, but rather to indicate what, as a result of the information discussed in the previous chapters, should be aimed for in a training schedule. We feel that it would be wrong for us to describe specific training schedules as we are not trainers ourselves. Rather we want to allow those readers who have already trained horses to be able to consider how they should modify their programmes as a result of the scientific information which is now available. When a leading exercise physiologist was asked prior to the last Olympic Games whether scientists would ever take over from coaches, he replied 'Scientists are interested in sports. They want to learn more about the function of the human body. They don't want to bother about becoming a coach as well.' In respect of the equine athlete, of course, the scientist is also directly concerned with helping in progress that is aimed at the welfare of the horse. The scientist's role is to work hand in hand with the coach or trainer, providing information on how they may best design the horse's training schedule.

In considering the design and functioning of a suitable training programme, there are three key words: 'specificity', 'individualism' and 'commonsense'. By specificity we mean that the type of fitness needed, and hence the training programme required, has to be related to the competition being aimed at. In other words, pure endurance training is of little use for a strength event such as a 5 or 6 furlong (1,000–1,200m) sprint. Likewise, short fast bouts of exercise will not get a horse fit for a 100 mile (161km) endurance ride. Individualism refers to the fact that every animal is different, and so an 'off the hook' training programme cannot be followed to the last letter, but has to be adjusted to the requirements of the individual horse and its responses. Although it is a good idea to have a structured training programme, this should be flexible enough to cater for each horse on a day-to-day basis. This leads to the last key word, commonsense, which is so important. One has to be able to assess when a horse is undergoing periods of overstress, leading to minor problems, and then to be able to take the appropriate action to modify the training programme and/or diet of the horse. This ability goes hand in hand with keen observation of the horse both at exercise and in the box or stall. Both the horse's mental attitude and its feeding habits should be noted, as well as any other changes. Such commonsense observation is often the key factor differentiating between a successful and an unsuccessful trainer.

One of the criticisms made of trainers, especially in the racing world, is that the time spent each day training a horse is very small compared with that spent by a human athlete. For example, in the USA where stables are located on the track, horses are only out for about half an hour per day, with training only involving perhaps one short burst of activity. It has been suggested, probably quite correctly, that such short brief bursts of training do not get the animal properly fit. It is also possible that such training is more likely to be successful at improving energy production than it is in developing desirable structural changes. There is, therefore, a greater liability to physical breakdown. Certainly, within the USA there is a very high incidence of breakdowns during the training of yearlings and the racing of two-year-olds, with large economic losses as a result. In the UK, training methods are slightly different, with horses being given longer periods of exercise, often being out for just over an hour. This extra time is not necessarily used for more speed work but allows more time for warming up and cooling down, both very important parts of a day's exercise. Whether racehorses would benefit from longer periods of exercise is currently under investigation by both researchers and trainers.

As has been pointed out on several occasions throughout this book, analogies cannot always be made from man to horse. There is also the point that it is not only quantity but also quality of training which counts, a point which is being appreciated by coaches of human athletes who are tending to move away from increasing even further the time spent on the track. Discussions on what constitutes an adequate amount of work to give a horse are not new. Even in Babylonian times there were trainers who worked horses either too hard or too little, as can be seen from the following quote from Daphne Machin Goodall's book, *A History of Horse Breeding* discussing training around 1300BC.

> Kikkukli's method of training covered exercise by day and night and included trotting and galloping over various differences, swimming, sweating, hot and cold bathing, and racing which lasted over several days and nights — a fairly exhausting sort of endurance test. The period of training covered 184 days.

Although researchers working with small groups of horses have been able to draw conclusions about the demands of different types of exercise on the horse, it is much more difficult, if not near impossible, for them to make definitive conclusions on the most appropriate training programmes for economic reasons. As will be appreciated by any horse owner today, the cost of keeping horses is extremely high and to carry out proper studies where one training programme is compared against another entails a minimum of twelve horses of similar age, ability and training status. Even if this were possible, injuries would tend to interfere with the design of the study and even result in the removal of animals. Another problem is that scientifically, all animals should be treated equally, thus removing any subjective bias, and this obviously goes against the earlier important consideration that each animal should be treated as an individual.

When considering the design of a training programme, the trainer has to decide in which area he is seeking an improvement. The relative importance of the particular areas will depend on the particular equestrian discipline being undertaken. So the trainer may be seeking:

1 Improved energy production to withstand fatigue.
2 Improvement in structure within the animal. Unfortunately, little is known about the feasibility of this.
3 Improved skill brought about by the developmnt of neuromuscular co-ordination.
4 Psychological familiarity leading to the animal carrying out the task in a relaxed manner which will lead to energy conservation.

The adaptations to the various body systems that will lead to improvements are summarised in Table 12.

Table 12 Training programmes are directed towards the following adaptations

1 Muscular	– a greater capacity for energy production
2 Cardiovascular	– increased heart size
	– increased capillary supply to muscle
	– increased blood volume

3 Lungs   –adaptations are unlikely, although some improve-
                         ment in gas transfer may occur as well as adaptation
                         of the respiratory muscles
4 Bone and tendon   – little known
5 Nervous system   – better integration for improved co-ordination in
                         events involving skill
                         – faster firing of nerves, allowing higher speeds
                         – psychological familiarity
6 Thermoregulation   – adaptations to heat

Obviously, all these factors are important, although in racing and endurance events factor 1 is very important, while it is less so in show-jumping and dressage, where factor 3 is of greater importance. As has already been described, movement depends on an increased generation of the high-energy compound, ATP. Depending on the intensity of the exercise being undertaken, very large amounts of ATP are required for sudden strenuous activities such as jumping, and for rapid acceleration. Continual physical activity, on the other hand, requires lower amounts of ATP but for a much more sustained period. In order to best achieve these differing requirements, different specific training regimes have to be employed. A similar situation is met when considering the differing requirements of power output.

In deciding what is the most appropriate training regime, it would obviously be useful to know what the metabolic requirements are for the different events. Unfortunately, little data is available on this subject in the horse, although recently a paper has been published giving an estimate of the contributions from aerobic and anaerobic metabolism in supplying ATP to the horse during various activities. It is interesting to compare this figure with the one given for man in Chapter 3. When results are compared for events lasting one or two minutes, it would appear that the contribution from anaerobic metabolism is greater in the horse than it is in man. Although it is known that the horse does have a greater capacity to produce lactate than man, it is likely that Table 13 overestimates the anaerobic contribution in the horse, especially that from phosphagens. The small amounts of phosphagens available in horse muscle can only contribute energy for a few seconds unless they are reformed via aerobic pathways. Whatever the exact contributions are, there is little doubt that during short periods of maximum exercise, the majority of the energy used comes from anaerobic metabolism. As will be illustrated later, there is probably little one can do to improve anaerobic metabolism but there is a great deal one can do to improve aerobic capacity. In fact, with horses racing over solely sprinting distances, we should be more concerned with developing power and co-ordination than with improving aerobic metabolism because, unfortunately, we cannot develop all three together.

Table 13   Estimates of relative contributions (%) of different sources of ATP to various equine activities

	Phosphagen	Anaerobic Glycolysis	Aerobic Metabolism
Showjumping	15	65	20
Polo	5	50	45
3-day event (cross-country)	10	40	50
Cutting events	88	10	2
Barrel racing	95	4	1
Racing			
Quarterhorses	80	18	2
Thoroughbreds: 1000m	25	70	5
1600m	10	80	10
2400m	5	70	25
3200m	5	55	40
Standardbreds: 1600m	10	60	30
2400m	5	50	45
Endurance	1	5	94
Pleasure and equitation show classes	1	2	97

(From Bayly W.M. in Exercise Physiology, The Veterinary Clinics of North America 1 (3) p599 W. B. Saunders Co. 1985)

One of the important considerations in training is to expose the body to similar stresses to those involved during competition so that suitable adaptations can occur. For example, if a horse is only trained at a slow canter, it may only have to recruit about 60 per cent of the fibres within a particular muscle. However, when a flat-out gallop is needed during a race 100 per cent of the fibres will have to be called upon. Naturally, the 40 per cent which have not previously been used cannot be expected to function as well as those which have been 'trained' and so they rapidly become fatigued.

This favourable effect of exposing tissues to the effects they are likely to endure during competition, thereby both increasing performance and reducing the risk of injury, is in line with the general theory of how the body adapts to stress. Training is, after all, just one of the many sources of stress to which an animal or man may be exposed during its life. The generally beneficial effects of stress were studied by a Canadian, Hans Seyle, who put forward the General Adaptation Syndrome Theory. This essentially says that when the body is exposed to an external stimulus that it has not previously adapted to, it will undergo changes that will allow it to withstand a similar stimulus or stress in the future. In terms of exercise, this means that various alterations, including those within the muscle, occur so that the body can better tolerate the next challenge. However, this adaptation does not always take place without problems to the animal. For example, if the stress is too great then immediate, possibly permanent, damage can occur, eg tendon sprains, fractures or even death. This situation is what animal welfare people and others refer to as stress, but really what they call stress is when overstress leads to distress. To reiterate, *stress* is a *beneficial* effect that is part and parcel of an adequate training programme, but for it to have its maximum beneficial effect without untoward harmful effects it has to be introduced using gradually increasing workloads and allowing sufficient recovery periods. Obviously, one cannot keep increasing the stress on the body indefinitely. As is well known to trainers, there comes a time when a peak effect is reached, and further work may actually result in a decline in the horse's fitness. This again fits in with Seyle's theory that you can overstress the system. As well as leading to other undesirable effects, these extra-stressful situations also make the animal more susceptible to any viral infections, etc, that might be around because the immune system becomes partially depressed. This probably explains why the greatest risk of respiratory infections occurs when animals are introduced to new stables and during times when their training is stepped up. The stress threshold will vary between different horses, another reason why each horse has to be treated as an individual.

Training programmes

So far, this chapter has dealt largely with the theory behind what should be aimed at in a training programme. Now we will describe how this may be put into practice. Any training programme consists of three basic parts as shown in Table 14.

Table 14   Training programme for optimum performance

1	Early stages	– low intensity exercise of moderate duration. To improve suppleness and joint mobility, adaptations to the saddle and the weight of the rider
2	Harder stages	– development of muscles and the cardiovascular systems either by continuous or interval training methods
3	Maintenance	– exercise that will allow the horse to maintain peak fitness. Will often involve a reduction in high intensity exercise, especially if competing regularly

1 **Early stages**   During the early stages, low-intensity exercise of moderate duration is undertaken, usually at the walk or light trot. This training will produce the early conditioning and will improve the

suppleness and mobility of joints and tendons. During this period much of the weight gained during the previous relative period of inactivity can be taken off as the horse is exercised for long distances at slow speed. It should be appreciated that the energy used while travelling any distance is very similar whether it is covered at a walk or gallop. So a 10 mile (16km) walk or trot will use ten times the energy of a 1 mile (1,600m) gallop. The time spent on training every day at this stage should ideally exceed an hour, with the time spent increasing as progress is made. In particular, the time spent trotting should be increased. The whole early stage should take at least one month, although this will depend on the prior training history of the horse. A longer period will be required for young animals coming into their first year of training, as not only will it help in conditioning but also in settling the horse into stable routine. As far as bringing about any adaptive changes in muscle and the cardiovascular system are concerned, little effect will be noted because during this stage of moderate activity only a small proportion of muscle fibres are recruited and the heart rates are unlikely to exceed 130–140 beats per minute. During this stage the horse does, however, become accustomed to carrying a saddle and rider, or in the case of trotters, pulling a cart (sulky). In summary, the importance of this stage is that it provides the foundation on which more intense workloads can be introduced.

2 **Harder stages**   The second stage is the period when real fitness is developed. It is also the time when specific training schedules are introduced aimed at the future competitive tasks. For instance, horses involved in activities based largely on strength, eg showjumping, cutting or quarterhorse racing, should have training incorporating basically anaerobic work and co-ordination in order to build up power. For the Standardbred trotter and middle distance, staying or jumping Thoroughbred, the programme has to consist of both power and aerobic elements. For endurance rides the object is to concentrate on training which will markedly increase the aerobic capacity and thus raise the anaerobic threshold. To accomplish any of these objectives a number of training programmes exist which involve either continuous or intermittent exercise schedules.

Training programmes based on continuous exercise are obviously used during the first stage of all training. For endurance training this type of training is continued in stage two, although with increasing fitness both the duration and the intensity are increased. It is suggested that, depending on the age and experience of the horse and the distance of the ride being aimed at, the horse should cover a distance of 96–193 miles (60–120km) per week. As the horse becomes fitter and the competition time gets nearer, a longer ride with distance and speed just under the ultimate aim should be undertaken. In the final two weeks before a ride the overall intensity of work is decreased, although one moderate length ride should be undertaken. During training for endurance rides, some high-intensity workouts are useful in order to improve the capacity to maintain high speeds and to increase the ability to move up steep hills. The best way to incorporate such high-intensity work into the training programme is with interval, or repetition, training, as will be described later.

Traditional methods of training Thoroughbred racehorses have also involved continuous training programmes. On fast work days the horses are briefly warmed up, given a short canter and then given a single bout of fast work (ie, ¾ speed or breezing) before being walked back to the stables. On slow work days, walking, trotting and slow cantering are performed over distances longer than the actual race distance. It should be noted that no top-class human athlete would use such a programme.

In an attempt to improve performance, some Thoroughbred racehorse trainers are now adopting intermittent training programmes. These have already been used for some time by trainers of eventers and trotters. The terms intermittent and interval training are essentially synonymous and refer to the horse undergoing a series of training bouts interspersed with periods of relief or recovery. The concepts and suggested advantages of interval training for the racehorse have been discussed at length by Tom Ivers in his book *The Fit Racehorse*. This details specific training schedules for Thoroughbred, Standardbred and Quarterhorse racing and is well worth reading by anyone interested in using interval training techniques. However, it should be appreciated that many of his ideas are controversial and have not yet been widely accepted by major trainers. As a result, it is a modification of true interval training which is generally used.

One of the biggest barriers to the general adoption of interval training is a lack of understanding of what it is. The term interval training does not imply anything about either the intensity or the duration of the workouts which the horse undertakes. In other words, the workload of each period of activity can vary from relatively easy, entirely aerobic exercise to high-intensity, largely anaerobic exercise. However, the workloads used are usually somewhere near the anaerobic threshold, ie the point at which energy production by the formation of lactic acid results in a marked build-up of this substance in the horse's blood.

The basic idea behind interval training is that it allows the horse to experience more intense work over the periods of activity than if the work was carried out in one continuous stretch. For example, you might be able to run several miles at ¾ or faster speed if it were to be broken up by relief periods, but you might not be able to run the same distance non-stop. By breaking the exercise up into segments, you are increasing the amount of high-intensity work that can be carried out, as well as avoiding marked signs of fatigue (and the undesirable physical and mental effects which can be associated with it). Working at these high intensities also requires the recruitment of a high percentage of the muscle fibres and lactic acid has to be produced to meet the energy requirements. You are, therefore, producing the stresses necessary to lead to favourable adaptation of the energy-generating systems in the muscles. The relief period which follows allows a partial recovery by removal of some of the lactic acid before the next exercise period. Normally, in training for middle- and long-distance events, the intensity of the work performed is only just above the anaerobic threshold in order to make sure that too much lactic acid is not produced. This may not be suitable for sprinters because it improves the aerobic capacity of the horse both by causing an increase in the number of capillaries supplying the muscle fibres and by increasing the amount of enzymes available to burn oxygen within the cells. The overall result is an increase in maximum oxygen consumption (VO_2 max).

When drawing up an interval-training programme, we use terms which are defined in Table 15. Although extensive guidelines are available for use in different human athletic fields, at the moment we are only in the formative years with regard to developing programmes for horses. As can be appreciated, large variations are possible in respect of the number of repetitions, the distances, the duration of the periods and their frequency. When a horse first starts on interval training, the time allowed for the work interval will be greater and the number of repetitions fewer than will be the case later on as fitness develops. To illustrate some of the present ideas on interval training for Standardbred and Thoroughbred horses, programmes described by an investigator at Washington State University are presented in Table 16 and 17. Here, the recovery time has been arbitrarily set at five minutes, and is spent at the walk. As can be seen from the tables, this worker considers that interval training should only be undertaken every four days because of the hard nature of this exercise and the need for full recovery afterwards. It should be appreciated that in deciding at which speed the horse should work, consideration has to be given to the fact that in racehorses especially the work rider is usually considerably heavier than the jockey carried during a race. So the desired effect can be obtained at less than racing speed. Whether more frequent high-speed workouts are desirable has to be investigated further. Obviously, on the days between these bouts of high-intensity work, lower intensity exercise is performed. At present, the programmes used in horses are adapted from man and use work periods of uniform intensity. In the Thoroughbred world these rigid programmes have been abandoned in favour of what might be considered a modified interval training. The actual work performed during the work periods then lies between that performed in the continuous programme described earlier and that of the fully structured interval training programme. So, after their warm-up period the horses are worked at increasing speeds but with rest periods in between each period of moderate to high-intensity exercise. Of course, interval training is not restricted to racehorses. It can be usefully incorporated as part of the training for the steeplechase and cross-country phases in eventing horses. For this type of activity, slightly longer work intervals at slower speeds would be used and, as well as the days devoted to slower work, time would also be devoted to training for the skills required in show-jumping and dressage.

Table 15   Definitions of terms related to interval training

Term	Definition
Work interval	That portion of the interval training programme consisting of the work effort — eg a 3f canter performed within a prescribed time.
Relief interval	The time between work intervals in a set. The relief intervals may consist of light activity such as walking (rest-relief) or mild to moderate exercise such as trotting (work relief).
Work-relief ratio	The time ratio of the work and relief intervals, eg a work-relief ratio of 1:2 means that the duration of the relief interval is twice that of the work interval.
Set	A group of work and relief intervals, eg four 3f canters (each performed within a prescribed time) separated by designated relief intervals.
Repetition	The number of work intervals per set.
Training time	The rate of work during the work interval.
Training distance	Distance of the work interval.
Frequency of training	Number of training sessions per week.
Session	A group of sets of repetitions.
ITP prescription	The specifications for the routines to be performed in a workout, eg: Set 1 $4 \times 3 @ 0.44 (3:00)$ where 4 = number of repetitions 3 = training distance in furlongs 0.44 = training time in minutes and seconds (3:00) = time of relief interval in minutes and seconds

Table 16   Sample interval training programme for Standardbred horses

Aim: Able to pace 1600m in 1:57 (1000m track).
Required base: At least 400km in previous 84 days.
Frequency: Every 4 days.
Relief-period criteria: HR 110 or less within 5 min of completing the interval. If not, session halted.
Interval criteria: If time greater than 1.5 sec outside scheduled time, session halted. Only proceed to next step if all criteria for previous level have been met.

Training level	Distance (m)	Number of heats	Time (min, sec)
1	600	2	0:56
2	800	2	1:15
3	1000	2	1:35
4	600	3	0:53
5	800	3	1:10
6	1000	3	1:28
7	1200	2	1:45
8	600	4	0:50
9	800	4	1:07
10	1000	4	1:25
11	1200	3	1:42
12	800	4	1:05
13	1000	4	1:23
14	1200	3	1:40
15	800	4	1:03
16	1000	4	1:20
17	1200	3	1:38
18	800	3	1:00
19	600	4	0:44
20	1000	2	1:18
21	800	2	0:58
22	600	3	0:42
23	1000	1	1:15
24	800	2	0.57
25	600	2	0:41

(From Bayly W.M. in Exercise Physiology, The Veterinary Clinics of North America 1 (2) p607 W. B. Saunders Co. 1985)

Table 17 Sample interval training programme for Thoroughbred horses

Aim: Successful racing over 1000 to 1400m.
Required base: At least 400km slow work over a minimum of 70 days.
Frequency: Every 4 days.
Relief-period criteria: HR 110 or less 5 min post interval, or session halted.
Interval criteria: If time more than 1.5 sec outside planned time, session halted. Do not proceed to next level until all criteria are met for previous step.

Training level	Distance (m)	Number of heats	Time (sec)
1	600	2	45
2	600	3	45
3	600	2	43
4	600	3	43
5	800	2	58
6	800	3	58
7	600	4	43
8	600	2	41
9	600	3	41
10	800	2	56
11	800	3	56
12	600	4	41
13	600	2	39
14	600	3	39
15	800	2	54
16	800	3	54
17	600	4	39
18	800	3	52
19	800	3	52
20	800	2	50
21	800	3	50
22	800	4	52
23	600	3	38
24	800	2	50
25	600	2	37
26	800	1	49
27	600	1	36
28	400	2	24

(From Bayly W.M. in Exercise Physiology, The Veterinary Clinics of North America 1 (3) p608 W. B. Saunders Co. 1985)

Rather than working to very precise times laid down in a book, which may have a varying effect on the horse, depending on the track and weather conditions (as well as on the horse's inherent ability), the effect of interval training can be assessed by using a heart-rate monitor. For example, initially it may be that one should aim at performing work which will result in heart rates of 180–200 beats per minute as these are around the anaerobic threshold level. With increasing fitness, higher work speeds can be used safely that produce heart rates above 200 beats per minute. The heart-rate monitors can also be used to monitor the recovery rate and so determine the duration of the recovery periods. Here the aim is partial recovery, around 110 beats per minute, rather than the 80 beats per minute usually found in a horse walking about before any exercise at all. If the heart rate ever exceeds what is expected for that particular stage of the programme, or it takes a prolonged time to fall back to the recovery levels, it is an indication that the exercise has become too stressful and no further work intervals should be undertaken. Unexpectedly, high heart rates during the warm-up or recovery periods may also be an early warning sign that all is not well with the horse because it has developed a low-grade lameness or, more rarely, an illness. A thorough examination of the horse should then be carried out.

Now that interval-training programmes have been described, their benefits and possible disadvantages can be outlined. Obviously, their main advantage is claimed to be that the horse becomes fitter, although it may take a longer period to achieve this end than with traditional training methods. The fitness is due to the development of the horse's aerobic metabolism so that not as much reliance is placed on the production of lactic acid. It is claimed, therefore, that horses will be better able to maintain their speed as they come down the finishing straight rather than slowing down as they might otherwise have done. It is also suggested that if a horse can withstand the stressful effects of the first few weeks of interval training, it is less susceptible to future musculo-skeletal injury. Survival of the fittest is not necessarily a bad thing for the future of the racing industry, but the ultimate aim must be to enable horses to race more frequently than would otherwise be possible and thus to increase the chances of the owner obtaining an economic return.

There are, however, a number of disadvantages and difficulties in putting a true interval-training programme into practice. Because it is a more time-consuming procedure than conventional programmes, it is more costly to the owner, although this will hopefully be repaid by better results. For best effect, it also requires good record-keeping. It may be that the chances of injury are greater during the earlier stages of interval training than during conventional training. However, this should only be the case if insufficient foundation work is carried out or if the horses are pushed too hard too early. People have questioned whether horses, especially the more highly strung Thoroughbreds, can psychologically tolerate programmes which only involve such short periods of maximum effort. It has, however, been found that young horses will adapt very well to interval training as long as it takes place away from large numbers of horses involved in more usual steady work. If anything, it may be more difficult to introduce the technique to older horses who have become set in their ways. One problem encountered in the USA, where horses are often trained on the same track where they subsequently have to race, is that during training, some horses may develop a habit of slowing down at certain parts of the track corresponding to the end of a work interval. Others may slow down completely as soon as the rider pulls on the reins.

One of the biggest problems associated with the incorrect use of interval training is that it could ruin a horse with good sprinting potential. It should be appreciated that the interval programmes so far discussed are essentially concerned with improving aerobic capacity and so developing stamina. Although this is desirable for endurance rides, eventing, middle- and long-distance racing, it could be detrimental to sprinting. This is because as the muscle cells change to increase their utilisation of oxygen, it is likely that many of the originally low oxidative fast twitch (Type IIB) fibres will alter in size. Now, originally these fibres have a larger cross-sectional area than the other types of fibres. However, as they become continuously called into use during the interval training, they need more oxygen. So, they actually decrease in size in order to allow easier movement of oxygen through the muscle cell. Unfortunately, power output is related to the size of the muscle mass contracting. The larger the muscle mass, the greater its potential power output. So, any reduction in muscle cell size will result in a smaller muscle mass and a reduced power output. This then reduces the ability for rapid acceleration and so there is a loss of sprinting ability. The importance of this muscle mass is readily seen if you look at the conformation of sprinters and stayers, whether human or equine. A sprinting horse will have a well-endowed, rounded gluteal muscle, whereas in the stayer and endurance horse it is much flatter. Studies in both man and laboratory animals have shown that it is not possible to develop both maximum strength and maximum stamina at the same time.

So what we need for the sprinting Thoroughbred or Quarterhorse is a training programme which places more emphasis on power (ie strength) than stamina. It is still possible to achieve this with a version of interval training interspersed with days of light work. In this case, the aim is only to bring the majority of the muscle fibres into play so that their aerobic capacity is not greatly increased. One of the main aims must be to improve neuromuscular co-ordination and even to increase the firing frequency of nerves so that rapid acceleration (and a speedy departure from the starting gate) can be produced. Sprint training involves repeated sprints at near-maximum speed but with complete recovery between each sprint. In this case, heart rate is allowed to recover to around 70 beats per minute, which may well take around ten minutes, depending on the horse's fitness. As can be seen from Table 13 such exercise involves the anaerobic system rather than developing the aerobic capacity. It is hoped that such power activities improve performance by increasing muscle mass as well as neuromuscular co-ordination. Repeated short bursts of activity, such as sprinting, for 1 furlong out of the starting gates, should improve the skill of rapid acceleration.

Another variation of interval training is repetition work, where the time spent on each work and relief period is steadily increased. Yet another variation is referred to as Fartlek training. This is really an unstructured training method carried out over variable terrain where slow and fast work are alternated. Generally, the fast work periods are kept well below maximum speeds and maintained as long as the horse does not tire. This type of training adds variety and helps to avoid boredom on the part of both the horse and rider. It is useful for endurance and eventing horses.

3 **Maintenance**   Once a horse has reached the desired level of fitness, the major problem is how to maintain this without any falling off in condition or the development of muscle or tendon injuries. Especially if the horse is competing at frequent intervals, the hard intensity workloads can be slightly reduced. This alone should be sufficient to maintain the strength and stamina of all the fast twitch fibres, but once again one has to consider the situation in each individual horse. It appears that the beneficial effects of training are not lost as quickly in the horse as they are in man. Their work capacity can survive several weeks of voluntary inactivity at the end of the season or involuntary inactivity as a result of injury, weather, etc.

There comes a point when further increased training may result in the condition of overtraining and reduced performance. Trainers often refer to a horse as being over-trained when explaining a poor performance, but whether and how this actually occurs is hard to tell. Certainly, such poor performance has been associated with an unusually high red blood cell mass (polycythemia) and a reduced level of cortisol production in the Standardbred, but we do not know whether the same applies to the Thoroughbred.

Skills

The importance of the development of skills in order to allow better and more efficient neuromuscular co-ordination has already been mentioned. Schooling for this co-ordination, whether for showjumping, dressage or leaving the starting gate, has to be included in every training programme. Even in endurance rides, the ability to maintain a relaxed temperament over even the most taxing of terrain has to be taught in order to conserve energy. We do not propose to venture into this field here; there are numerous books available describing how various competitors undertake the teaching and development of these skills.

Warming up and cooling down

A satisfactory warming-up period before and a cooling-down period afterwards are integral parts of training programmes at all three stages. Obviously, the aim is to reduce the risk of injuries during and following exercise. An adequate period of walking and trotting not only loosens up the muscles and tendons but also, by increasing the blood supply to the muscles, prepares them for the marked increase in metabolic demands which result from fast work. This low level of muscular activity and associated increase in blood supply results in a slight rise (about 1.8°F (1°C)) in muscle temperature. The higher temperature is beneficial for two reasons. A higher temperature increases enzyme activity and it also appears to improve muscle contractions and reflex times. A warming-up period is just as important for short sprint activities where sudden acceleration without prior warming up can lead to tearing of the muscle fibres. Another important function of the warming-up period is that it allows the rider or trainer to spot any minor lamenesses. If there is time before starting the walking, some stretching exercise can be carried out. This involves picking up each leg and then flexing and extending the entire limb upwards and downwards, forwards and back. It is suggested that this should be repeated eight to ten times for each leg.

Cooling down should be carried out in the reverse order to warming up, ie trotting before walking. Despite the use of the word 'cooling', a lowering of temperature is not the main aim of this period. One of the favourable effects of a cooling-down period after strenuous exercise is that it speeds up the washing out of lactic acid from the muscles and the bloodstream. The effects of different types of activity during the cooling-down period after strenuous exercise which produced high levels of lactate is shown in Fig 36. As well as helping in the removal of lactate,

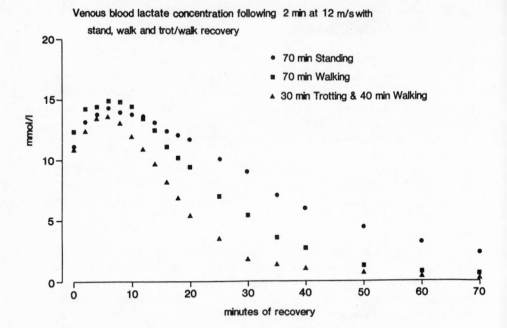

Fig 36 The rate of lactate removal from the muscle and blood is increased by light activity after maximal effort

slow trotting also stimulates a more rapid recovery of the phosphagen stores. So, in interval training it is probably better to trot the horse slowly during the recovery period than just to walk because this will result in a more complete recovery. Following the cooling-down period, the horse is than returned to its stable where further cooling and washing may take place.

'Up hill and down dale'

Working horses up and down hills has several advantages. As horses cannot be trained to lift weights, other than those carried on their backs, they cannot use weight-lifting to improve their power as human sprinters do. Some trainers are experimenting to see whether pulling weights while working, even as yearlings, may result in muscle developments similar to weight-lifting. When horses run up a hill, however, they have to accelerate continually in order to overcome the continuing slope. The effect is similar to weight-lifting. This sort of work, therefore, is extremely good at building up the strength of certain muscle groups in both the front and back legs. The other advantage is that the same physical effort can be obtained at a slower speed up-hill than it can over flat ground. This results in lower concussive forces on the joints, but an increased load in the tendons. Hill training is used extensively in the UK. Even at Newmarket, the so-called 'home of flat racing', one can see hundreds of horses every day running up the relatively steep incline of Warren Hill (see plate 21).

Training young horses

In addition to looking at the effects of training methods on horses aged two years old and upwards, investigations are also being made into the desirability of using some form of training in yearlings. For example, exercising on a treadmill may help muscle development without imposing undue stress on the immature skeletal system.

Training aids

A variety of ancillary equipment is being introduced to training establishments both for economic reasons as labour becomes more expensive, and to reduce boredom or to help in rehabilitation after injury. Such equipment must remain an accessory to normal training methods; it obviously cannot replace normal track work.

Horse walkers have found wide popularity in the USA and Australia, but are much less common in Britain. They are probably of little use in cardiovascular or muscular development but can provide the light exercise necessary during warming-up and cooling-down periods. Their main benefit is on economic grounds, as a number of horses can be exercised at the same time with virtually no manpower.

Treadmills have also found fairly wide popularity, although not nearly as great as the horse walker. Early treadmills were only capable of work at the walk or slow trot, although some compensated for this by having inclines of 20° or more. These treadmills were generally poorly built, made a lot of noise when running and had surfaces which became slippery when covered in sweat. Although they had their uses, overall, they were far from satisfactory. Commercially manufactured high-speed treadmills, based on the one that has been in operation for almost twenty years in the Veterinary School in Sweden, have recently been made in Sweden and Australia. (Plate 22). These allow horses to be exercised safely at speeds in excess of 30mph (50kmph) and as they can be inclined up to 10°, work efforts similar to those experienced during racing can be achieved, ie heart rates in excess of 200 beats per minute. It is amazing how quickly horses can become accustomed to exercising on these treadmills, even at fast gallops. It has been found that even horses which are difficult to ride can be exercised in this way without becoming sour. For safety reasons, horses should always wear a harness in case the treadmill should inadvertently stop at high speed owing to a power cut, etc. In addition to their use in research units, some treadmills have been bought by trainers. Although the advanced models cost around £20,000–25,000 compared with £4,000–5,000 for the earlier models, their greater versatility and safety would fully justify the difference where expensive horses are involved. Besides being used as a training aid prior to racing, they may also be useful in maintaining fitness in horses which have back problems because the horse can be exercised without a rider on its back. Another circumstance in which they have been used is to give horses hard workouts when either weather or other ground conditions do not permit normal work. In the near future we should be able to form a better opinion of the everyday use of such machines. In the veterinary field it may well be that they will be of great assistance in investigating exercise-related problems, whether in the cardiac, respiratory, muscular or skeletal systems.

Swimming has been used for a long time as a training aid, although its usefulness has long been debated by trainers. (Plate 23). Some believe that swimming can do a lot of good but others think it is of little benefit. Where stables are near water, their horses can naturally swim there, otherwise special pools have to be built. These are generally circular, with special ramps leading in and out of the water. A study of swimming by a group of Japanese workers found that the horse kicks out harder with the outside leg when swimming round in a circle, so horses using a circular pool regularly should go in both directions to prevent abnormal muscle development. Despite this, some trainers who only swim their horses in one direction have found no problems. Most horses take readily to swimming. As can be appreciated from a look at the heart rates of swimming horses, it is a strenuous type of exercise that is suitable for both developing muscle and improving cardiopulmonary function. During free swimming, heart rates will range from 140 to 170 beats per minute. An even greater effort can be achieved by making the horses swim against a current.

Swimming is extremely useful in horses suffering from joint and tendon problems as it keeps the weight off their joints and legs. It is also useful in maintaining fitness in horses that are prone to jarring. Another use of swimming is as a form of different exercise to relieve boredom in horses that may have soured of normal training methods. Once again, however, it cannot replace normal training methods. A routinely high component of swimming in a training programme would only be useful if swimming races existed for horses!

Recently, a device has been built which is a cross between a flat treadmill and a pool of water. The idea behind this water treadmill is that rather than using swimming, which may result in unnatural muscle development, the horse actually walks and trots in water up to its belly. The water introduces an extra workload which the horse has to overcome, but it also acts as a cushion against the concussive effects of landing on the limbs. From measurements using heart-rate meters, the workload is not very great, as heart rates rarely exceed 100 beats per minute. Again, the main usefulness of this machine may lie in the rehabilitation of horses after injury and possibly in the early training of young horses.

Assessment of fitness

The end result achieved from a training programme will depend on both the horse's inherent performance capacity and its state of fitness. The horse's inherent ability includes factors which are fixed at birth for that horse, such as its constitution. These are the endogenous factors over which the trainer has no control. There are also, however, exogenous or external factors, such as diet and degree of training. These will determine whether the inherent ability of the horse can be fully expressed. In the final analysis, it is only during an actual competition that we can see how these factors have influenced performance. Nevertheless, attempts have been made to measure both the potential and fitness of horses before they reach the day of the competition. Some of the tests used for this purpose will be considered in more detail.

We are obviously aiming all the time at achieving full fitness, ie developing the required skills for a particular task so that the animal can run faster or for longer periods without the onset of fatigue. The fitness requirements will differ with the level of competition, and one of the difficulties is being able to judge exactly when the appropriate stage of fitness has been reached. Most riders and trainers have their own set of criteria for deciding this, based on their own past observations. Such a system of evaluation is too individual, and will vary too much from trainer to trainer, to be of value scientifically. For the true evaluation of different training programmes, or for the clinical assessment of horses suspected of having problems causing impaired performance, more precise measurements are necessary. In recent years, some of the fitness tests which have been developed in the human athlete have been adapted and evaluated in the horse. As well as being sophisticated enough to give precisely measurable results, the test must also be capable of being reproduced by people working in different countries, etc. Standardised exercise tests allow comparisons to be made both for a particular animal at varying stages of its training programme and between different animals at the same stage of training. The latter therefore provides a measure of their relative abilities. The tests have been designed to evaluate the muscular, cardiovascular and respiratory systems. In man tests have been devised to assess both strength and stamina, but so far we have only developed tests of stamina, ie aerobic capacity, in the horse.

Fitness has physical, mental and health aspects, and any of these may interfere with performance. We are concerned mainly with the question of investigating physical fitness. In the past, books on training have tended to ignore this question of assessing fitness. It has been implied that if you follow such and such a training programme the horse will automatically get fit. This is by no means the case in practice, however. Even the very best trainers, who have no difficulty in assessing general competitive fitness, will admit that there may be difficulties in assessing particular horses.

Observation
Keen observation is the method of fitness assessment most relied upon. This involves the trainer depending upon his knowledge of the horse and how it has responded to similar workloads in the past. The rider and trainer have to rely mainly on observing changes in the horse's gait to indicate the onset of fatigue. In addition, the sounds of its breathing, and the character of that breathing, give some indication of the respiratory effort which has been involved, especially immediately after a work-out when an unfit horse takes more frequent forced expirations than a fit horse. This is because the unfit horse has produced more lactic acid and therefore needs more oxygen to burn it off. It will also produce more carbon dioxide after the exercise has finished.

In some countries respiratory rates are used as one of the criteria in assessing whether a horse should be allowed to continue an endurance ride after the mandatory stops. In the USA and Australia, although respiratory rates are noted, high rates do not result in the horse being eliminated. In the UK, however, if the respiratory rate climbs to twice the heart rate after a thirty-minute stop, then the horse is eliminated. It has been argued, with much justification, that respiratory rates should not be used for this purpose as they may not indicate a fatigued horse. Increased respiratory rates can occur, for example, in horses that are using panting as a means of helping to dissipate heat. This is especially common in rides held in hot conditions, when a fast, shallow respiration is often seen. It is only when respiration is both frequent and deep in character that fatigue should be suspected. In these cases the heart rate should also be raised.

Timing

Obviously one of the best methods to assess any improvement is by timing the horse working over a given distance. This is used in many countries where training is carried out on the racecourse. To be meaningful, daily variations in track conditions have to be taken into account, and the same rider/driver used. In the UK timing is infrequently used, as training is carried out over different gallops. Instead progress is judged by how a horse works against another of equal ability.

Weight

Another aid to assessing fitness is the horse's weight. As most horses enter training overweight, a reduction should occur with training as the A in fAtness is turned to the I in fItness. Although it would appear obvious that an overweight fat horse or human cannot perform at its best, it is surprising how many horses appear overweight at both the racetrack and at other forms of competition. Often the reason for this is that the owner/trainer wants the horse to appear in good condition and not as skin and bones. It should be realised that an overweight horse is handicapped just as much as if it were carrying an overweight rider, and this applies to any event that involves maximum effort, whether race or endurance ride. This is because the more weight that is carried, the more energy has to be used per stride when the horse has to raise itself above the ground. Although we have suggested that fat is a very important fuel for energy during long-term exercise, this is no justification for competing with a fat horse, as even the leanest horse has more than enough supplies of fat. One has only to look at successful long-distance runners of both the human and equine variety to see that they are all lean and do not carry any surplus weight.

Although there are many riders and trainers who claim that they can accurately estimate a horse's weight, and small changes in it, by eye, when they are put to the test they are usually inaccurate. The best way of following any weight changes is by using one of the commercially available walk-on weighbridges. Alternatively, the weight can be estimated from measurements:

$$\text{Weight of the horse in lb} = \frac{G^2 \times L}{300}$$

where G is the girth measured in inches just behind the elbow and L is the length in inches from the point of the withers to the tuber ischii (a bony prominence just to the side of the tail).

A number of the leading racing stables in Britain have found from weighing their horses that each horse has an ideal racing weight. What is, perhaps, even more surprising is that the racing authorities pay little attention to any marked fluctuations in the racing weights of horses. In greyhound racing, on the other hand, unless the dog is within a narrow range on either side of its declared racing weight, it will not be allowed to run. This is done to try to prevent inconsistent performances due to running fat dogs or dogs which have been given a very large feed just prior to racing. Within the horse-racing world, it is only in Japan and a few other minor racing countries that the weighing of horses on race days is undertaken. Some trainers even weigh their horses before they leave for and after they return from the racecourse. This helps them to assess how much stress the race has imposed on the horse. As would be expected, it has been found that some horses regularly lose more weight during a race than others. Perhaps surprisingly, a horse's ideal racing weight does not alter between its two- and three-year-old seasons.

Table 18 Examples of similar ideal racing weights in 2- and 3-year old Thoroughbreds (taken at time of winning)

	Weight(kg)	
Horse	2yr	3yr
1	414	416
2	394	390
3	440	442
4	518	518
5	520	520
6	422	420
7	464	466

(Results courtesy of C. Brittain, Newmarket)

Assessing aerobic capacity

As we have explained, increasing stamina or endurance ability depends on increasing the horse's aerobic capacity. This in turn increases the anaerobic threshold so that higher speeds can be undertaken before lactic acid is produced and builds up. At the same time, more energy can be produced from burning fat rather than glucose. A number of methods, of varying complexities, have been devised to measure any improvement in aerobic capacity. The tests can be carried out either on a high-speed treadmill or in the field. The most reproducible results are obtained on the treadmill because then the speed, going and weather conditions can be kept constant.

Oxygen consumption

In man, one of the oldest methods of measuring improved aerobic capacity was to measure changes in maximal oxygen consumption (VO_2 max) during the training programme. The tests were carried out either on a treadmill or on a bicycle ergometer. However, this test is not as frequently used today as an aid to measuring improved fitness as it used to be. This is because the differences between individual performances are largely genetically determined, and only surprisingly small increases occur with training, despite an obvious increase in fitness. In horses determination of the VO_2 max is only in its infancy, although horses will tolerate wearing the masks necessary for these tests. It is unlikely that this particular test will come into routine use for measuring fitness in horses, despite its use in assessing performance potential in man.

Anaerobic threshold

As the determination of VO_2 max has fallen out of favour, so the measurement of the anaerobic threshold has increased in popularity. This involves finding the workload at which there is a sudden upsurge in the amount of lactic acid in the blood, ie finding the point when production in the muscle is not matched by the rate of its removal from the blood. The anaerobic threshold is obtained by working the individual at a number of speeds for two or three minutes per workload, and taking blood samples each time for lactate determination. The results are then plotted on a graph and the anaerobic threshold determined. For ease of working, this point is now usually considered to be when blood lactate exceeds 4m mol/litre. In both the scientific and popular press the anaerobic threshold is also referred to as the Onset of Blood Lactate Accumulation (OBLA). In man, there is a very close correlation between anaerobic threshold and performance in marathon races. The higher the anaerobic threshold, the faster the marathon can be run. Over shorter distances, however, especially middle-distance events, there is not such a good correlation. A number of research groups are trying to evaluate anaerobic threshold as a means of assessing fitness and performance in horses. The horses can be worked for two minutes on a treadmill at a number of progressively increasing speeds, or they can be exercised over 1,090yd (1,000m) at each of four different speeds. An example of a test reading for a Standardbred is given in Table 19.

Table 19   Example of a standardised exercise test and expected heart rates in Standardbred horses

	Speed (yd (m)/min)	Heart rate (beats/min)
Step 1	490–600 (450–550)	170–180
Step 2	680–765 (600–700)	190–200
Step 3	765–875 (700–800)	210–120
Step 4	>875 (>800)	>220

(From Wilson and others, in *Equine Exercise Physiology*, p488, Granta Editions, Cambridge, 1983)

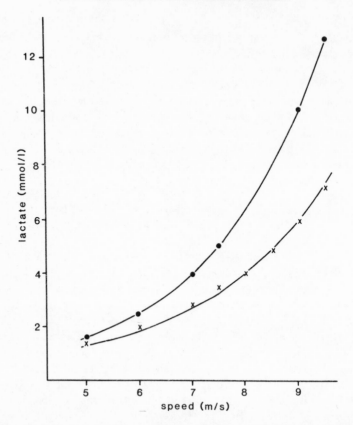

Fig 37 The effect of training on the anaerobic threshold (i.e. with rise in blood lactate concentration). Note the higher speed with training before the increase in blood lactate. (Adapted from Thornton and others in *Equine Exercise Physiology*, p.481, Granta Editions, Cambridge, 1983)

As can be seen from Fig 37, increasing fitness results in an increasing anaerobic threshold. It has also been found that within Standardbred trotters of similar training status, distinct groups existed. Those with the higher anaerobic thresholds were the best performers. Whether such a test would be of any use in Thoroughbreds is still being evaluated, although here the reduced strength which follows greater oxidative capacity may be a disadvantage.

Plate 18 Endoscopy in a horse

Plate 19 A scanning electron microscope picture of the cells found lining the smaller airways. Note, some have thin finger-like projections (cilia) which are very important in removing debris from the airways. (Photograph courtesy K. Whitwell)

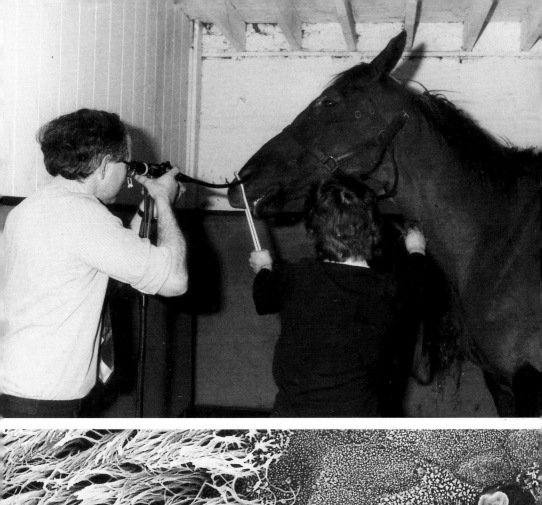
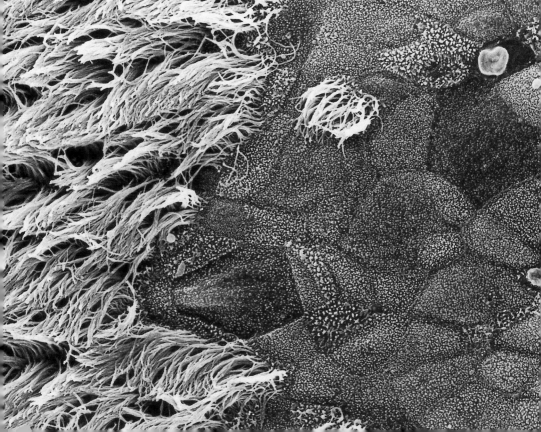

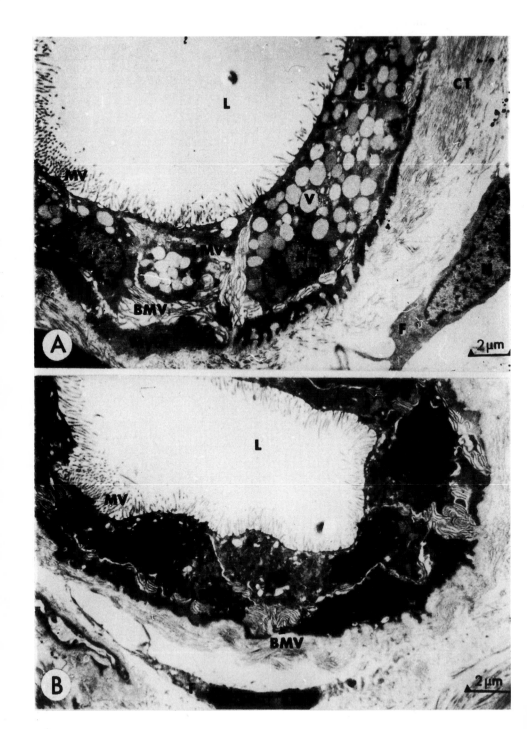

Heart rates

Of all the objective means of assessing fitness, measuring the heart rate is the easiest to do, and can be readily carried out by moŝt owners and trainers. To this end a number of on-board heart-rate monitors are available to measure heart rates during both exercise and recovery. Their use has been discussed in Chapter 5.

When horses are worked at the same effort and the same level of fitness, reproducible heart rates are obtained. Work effort is not, however, the only factor which can increase heart rate. External stimuli which cause apprehension and anxiety will also have this effect, especially at low workloads. For example, a working heart rate of 120 beats per minute may suddenly rise to 180 beats per minute for a short time if the horse is startled. Using increasing workloads, it has been shown that the heart rate increases steadily between 120 and 210 beats per minute. Above this level, however, there is a plateau effect (Fig 38). As horses become fitter, it is generally agreed that their resting heart rates become slower.

It has been suggested that one way to assess fitness is to measure the speed of exercise needed to cause a heart rate of 200 beats per minute. This particular heart rate is chosen as representing the VO_2 max of the horse. In one treadmill study in standardbreds it was found that after five weeks training, the VO_2 max had increased from 8.04 to 8.7yd (7.35 to 7.96m) per second on a 10 per cent slope. Incidentally, this speed is not arrived at by adjusting the treadmill speed until a heart rate of 200 beats per minute is reached but by using increasing speeds to find the precise VO_2 max. Some differences in heart rate response between unfit and fit horses are shown in Fig 38. Standardbreds are often used in such tests because their speed is easily regulated and they maintain a constant pace.

Besides measuring the heart rate during exercise, it is also useful to monitor it during recovery. The most rapid fall in heart rate occurs in the first few minutes after exercise. When using recovery heart rates to assess fitness, it has been found that the rate five minutes after exercise is the most useful. In general during endurance rides, a heart rate below 60 beats per minute is required (measured thirty minutes after arrival at the compulsory stop) before the horse is allowed to continue.

Plate 20 Electron microscope picture of the sweat forming part of the sweat gland a) shortly after the commencement of sweating, b) after 4 hours sweating. Note the disappearance of the vesicles and flattening of the cells in b). V = secretory vesicles (probably containing protein. L = lumen of gland. MV = microvilli into lumen. BMV = basal microvilli. (Photograph courtesy I. Montgomery)

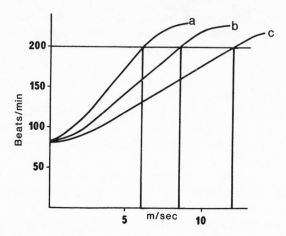

Fig 38 The effects of training and disease on heart rate response to exercise. Note that over most of the heart rate range there is a linear increase related to the exercise intensity. At high work rates there is a plateauing of heart rate. A) cardio-circulatory disorder, B) moderately fit, C) endurance trained. (Adapted from SGB Persson in *Equine Exercise Physiology*, p442, Granta Editions, 1983)

Lameness can also affect heart rate before it even becomes visible to an observer. This is because lameness requires an increased effort from healthy legs. This kind of early warning information can only be obtained, however, if daily monitoring is carried out.

Enzymes
The monitoring of enzymes that may indicate muscle damage can also be useful in assessing fitness. In the early stages of training, when heavier workloads are first introduced, elevations in the levels of creatine phosphokinase (CPK) and aspartate aminotransferase (AST or GOT) often occur due to muscle damage. With increasing fitness, however, these changes disappear, until in fit racehorses remarkably constant values are seen week after week. When this state is reached, even a small increase in enzyme levels should be investigated as potentially significant. In endurance horses, on the other hand, the enzymes can be high even before the event and the horse will still compete successfully. We do not know how they manage to do this.

Assessment of health
Increasing physical fitness is worthless unless it goes hand in hand with physical health. Health assessment is at its most accurate when it is backed up by careful observation of the horse at work and at rest. Factors such as proper worm control and vaccination programmes are

obviously important. Similarly, we all know that without a good foot there cannot be a good horse, so proper shoeing is important, although it is often not achieved even in the racing world where stud values of millions of pounds may hang on the performance of those feet on the track. The key person in the health sphere is the veterinary surgeon. Some trainers get their veterinary surgeon to carry out regular blood monitoring of their horses. This involves both red and white cell counts, etc. If such monitoring is to be of any use in the early detection of problems, samples must be taken at least every month during the training/performing season. Further samples will be needed at times of peak concern or stress. Only in this way can proper base-line values be worked out for each individual horse. Changes in a horse's blood cells may only be slight but may still be important. Without a proper base-line we cannot place sufficient importance on these small changes. For once, the attention given by many trainers to the health of their horses, including blood checks, etc, is in sharp contrast to the situation in human athletes. In Britain, for example, little attention is directed towards monitoring the health of even our international athletes. This is one area (and perhaps the only one) where the equine world is ahead of its human counterpart.

9 · Feeding for Performance

Throughout this book, reference has been made to the various 'fuels' which the different body systems require. Such has been the growth of interest in human diets over the last couple of decades that everyone is now familiar with the fact that the diet of any mammal, be it man or horse, must contain a balance of ingredients. These may be grouped together as carbohydrates, fats, proteins and essential vitamins and minerals. Before considering the feedstuffs themselves, it is necessary to understand exactly how the horse's digestive system works.

The grazing horse
The horse is basically a grazing animal. It is unnatural for it to be given any food other than free-range grazing. Every time we fill a horse's feed bucket we are departing from nature. Even hay can be said to be an unnatural food when it is being fed as the sole roughage. It is true that the horse turned out in a field during the autumn and winter will eat a lot of dried herbage which is similar to, but probably not as high quality nutritionally, as hay, but it will still be eating 'wet' green food as well.

The horse grazes by biting off the grass with its incisor teeth, the teeth across the front of its mouth. If there is no contact between the upper and lower incisors, it will be a very inefficient grazer. The most common situation where this occurs is when the horse is 'parrot mouthed', ie when its upper jaw is too long and the upper incisor teeth are so far in front of the lower incisors that they do not make contact. As long as there is any appreciable contact, however, the horse will be able to graze normally. The fact that a horse is slightly over-shot, with the front edge of its upper incisors slightly in front of the lower ones, would not affect the decision whether to buy a competition horse. The horse prefers to graze short rather than long grass, and once it has been cut by the incisors, chewing is aimed at bruising the plant material to allow the juices to escape and the horse's digestive juices to have better access to the material which has to be digested, rather than at cutting the fibrous material into shorter lengths. It follows that when we provide hay as the basic roughage ration, the incisors have no cutting action but merely grasp the strands of hay to help get them into the mouth. The molar, or chewing, teeth then have a much harder material to deal with. They have almost to shred the hay so that it can be digested, but this does not necessarily cut it into shorter lengths. The result is that although grass and hay are digested in basically similar ways and contain similar ingredients, the fibrous material in hay is of a much greater length and this may present problems.

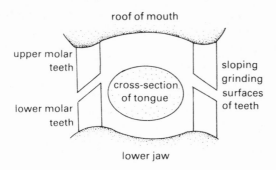

Fig 39 Tooth wear: cross section of the mouth showing tongue and teeth on either side

The mechanics of eating

The vast majority of athletic horses will be receiving supplementary food as well as roughage. This will require grinding by the molar teeth no matter whether it has been fed as a coarse ration or as a commercial pellet. The action of the horse's jaws means that chewing wears away a sloping table of wear on the molar teeth (Fig 39). This produces two self-sharpening edges, one on the outside of the upper teeth and the other on the inside of the lower teeth. There comes a point at which the discomfort produced by the movement of these sharp points discourages the horse from chewing more than the absolute minimum, which may not be sufficient to allow efficient digestion of the food. The more supplementary food you require the horse to consume to fuel its performance, the more critical this efficiency of chewing becomes. It follows that where a horse is being asked for maximum performance, regular dental care is essential to ensure both reliable response to the bit and efficient food digestion. Apart from the question of dental problems, it is not necessarily a good thing for a horse to finish all its food quickly. A slower rate of eating may improve digestibility and reduce boredom. The addition of chaff (chopped hay or straw) to the diet can improve protein and fibre digestibility, and so improve their nutritional value, by slowing the rate of consumption.

An interesting fact about the horse is that it only salivates during the time that it is actually chewing; it cannot moisten its mouth at will in the same way as we can. Horses which have been severely stressed will sometimes stand playing with a wisp of grass or hay in their mouth solely in order to stimulate salivation and moisten the mouth. This is almost invariably seen, for instance, when a horse has recovered from a general anaesthetic and is keen to get rid of that dry mouth which those people who have had an anaesthetic will remember so well. The practice of sponging a horse's mouth out with fresh water during the break between the roads and tracks section and the cross-country section of a horse trials, for instance, is thus well based on scientfic knowledge.

The digestive processes
Digestion of the horse's food is very much bound up with the anatomy of its digestive tract. The food passes from the mouth down the oesophagus to the stomach, with the salivary enzymes already in action. The stomach is relatively small in capacity because in nature, as has been mentioned, it only has to cope with a more or less continuous slow supply of roughage. When we decide to give supplementary feeds, we must appreciate that it is much more efficient to double the number of feeds than it is to double the amount of food fed on each occasion. No system works at its best when it is being pressed at maximum capacity, and the digestion of carbohydrates in the horse's stomach is no exception. A regular stable routine also helps to ensure that maximum food value is obtained with minimum risk of digestive upset.

After leaving the stomach, the food passes into the small intestine, which occupies much of the space in the upper abdomen. Here, digestion of soluble carbohydrates (or starches) which are largely responsible for restoring glycogen in muscle, and proteins occurs, especially the higher quality proteins. In the human being this completes the digestion, and when the material passes on to the large colon, all that remains is to reabsorb much of the moisture and electrolyte content to avoid the loss of too much fluid. In the horse, however, there is the problem of what to do with the relatively indigestible fibre and cellulose which makes up so much of its roughage diet. The solution has been to increase the capacity of the large colon, which lies like two interconnecting U shapes (Fig 40) in the abdomen. Millions of 'friendly' bacteria of many different types are allowed to live, multiply and die here because they live off the undigested fibre. The result of all this activity is that this living soup becomes rich in simple types of carbohydrates, volatile fatty acids (one of which when absorbed is rapidly converted to glucose), and proteins, which the walls of the large colon can readily absorb into the horse's own

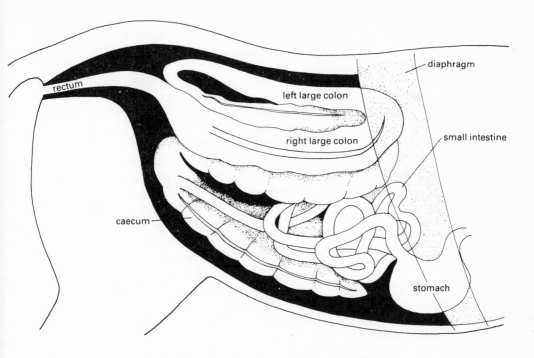

Fig 40 Schematic diagram of the digestive system of the horse

bloodstream. The only disadvantage is that each type of bacteria is relatively specific over the particular foodstuff which it will digest. As long as we feed the horse a constant ration, the numbers of bacteria will adjust themselves so that they are present in the ideal proportions to cope with the food they are presented with. Any sudden change in diet, even one as slight as changing the source of the hay, will require a different proportion of bacterial types. If the bacteria cannot adapt quickly enough, then the fibre will not be digested and may literally bung up the system by accumulation thus causing an intestinal impaction.

Colic
Horses which are competing and in full training may, to some extent, 'live on their nerves'. All their body systems are under some degree of extra stress, and even relatively minor changes in their routine may disrupt their digestive pattern. When such a horse gets an attack of colic (colic being defined as abdominal pain), it is difficult to determine whether it is the nervous control of the alimentary tract which has become upset, or whether it is the passage of food, etc along the tract which has affected the whole system. The important thing is that the

normal peristalsis, as we call the alternate waves of contraction and re-laxation rhythmically passing along the bowels, is interrupted. When this happens, some areas of the bowel will become distended and stretched more than normal. It is this stretching (rather than any of the contractions) which is painful and causes the symptoms of colic.

So horses which have travelled for longer distances than normal, or which are being stabled in strange surroundings and under unfamiliar routines prior to a competition, may develop an acute colic just at the time when one least wants it. The colic itself will obviously need treat-ment, but the drugs which are used may well render the horse liable to disqualification because they are not permitted under the competition rules. For this reason, some people have been known to delay treatment in the hope that the problem will disappear spontaneously. Ethically, there can be little justification for allowing the horse to continue to suf-fer pain for such a reason. Treatment of such acute colic may involve the use of analgesics or various forms of sedative/muscle-relaxant drugs. Some of these will be discussed in Chapter 10. The trend has been to develop drugs which have a long period of activity, whereas in this par-ticular situation the ideal would be a drug with a short period of action but which was then rapidly eliminated from the horse's body. It might also be worth pointing out that the horse may cause physical damage to itself during an attack of colic, eg muscular bruising, which may not be immediately obvious. Prompt treatment of the colic may rule out the im-mediate competition but safeguard future performance.

Feeding for energy

Providing the correct amount of energy is perhaps the most difficult problem in feeding the athletic horse. A resting, stabled, 880lb (400kg) adult horse needs 50 megajoules (MJ) of digestible energy every day, digestible energy being the amount of energy which the horse can actu-ally obtain from the food rather than the theoretical maximum that could be obtained. This requirement goes up to 69MJ per day for a 1,100lb (500kg) horse and to 79MJ for a 1,320lb (600kg) horse. The first point to note here is that a horse 50 per cent heavier does not need 50 per cent more energy per day, but only just over 35 per cent more. The other point is that these are values for mature horses. The requirements of competing animals and for growing animals, eg a two-year-old racehorse, will be even higher. Although the energy requirements in-crease appreciably with activity, very little work has been carried out to determine what the exact energy requirements are. This is especially the case for the horse at high-intensity work, where it is now thought that energy requirements are about 20-30 per cent higher than previously thought. From an evaluation of the diet at a Thoroughbred stable in Britain it was found that during the period of intense training and/or racing, approximately 210MJ of digestible energy was fed per day, while during early training it was 160MJ. In contrast, surveys on race-tracks in North America have shown that approximately 150MJ per day of digestible energy was being fed. As it can be assumed that in all instances the horses were in racing condition, this gives a good guideline to the energy requirements. The lower energy requirements in the American horses is probably due to the fact that their period of work per day is about half that of the British. In Standardbreds, the daily requirement in training is approximately 155MJ.

In horses in extensive training for endurance competitions it is likely that the energy requirements are even higher, and this might lead to a problem in providing sufficient energy. This is because the maximum dry matter consumption is about 2.5-3.0 per cent of its body-weight. In other words, a 880lb (400kg) endurance horse can eat only about 26lb (12kg) of feed on a dry-matter basis per day. Therefore, to meet the high-energy requirements for such activities without overloading the digestive system, fats can be fed.

Many horse owners are so worried about under-feeding and not providing sufficient energy that they over-feed. This is especially likely with inexperienced owners during the last few days prior to an event. The problems of over-feeding often only become evident with exercise, when azoturia occurs. Over-feeding is less likely to be a problem in competition horses, because they will be burning off a lot of the energy. This does not necessarily mean, however, that the horse will always be receiving enough energy. Dental problems, as have been mentioned, high parasite levels and poor food absorption can all mean that an adequate ration does not provide sufficient energy for the consumer, the athletic horse.

The main sources of energy in a horse's diet are the various cereals and the hay. In this respect we are treating grass as a superior form of hay because the comments on the constituents of hay apply just as well to the grass, except that an owner can go out onto the open market and buy hay of any kind he likes or can afford, whereas he is stuck with the grazing he has and cannot usually change it. The best source of energy is sugar because this gives 16MJ per 2.2lb (kg), but there is a limit to the number of sugar-lumps you should give a horse. People often claim that a particular food source makes their horse 'hot' and difficult to control, or that another makes it fat. These are not really differences in the type of energy provided but more differences which arise owing to the concentration of digestible energy in a given weight of the food or to variations in the weight of the food which fills a given volume. Energy levels are worked out by weight, and the weight of particular food which will fill the horse's small stomach may be very different from the weight of another food which it can eat in the same time.

Table 20   The digestible energy content of cereals

Grain	Digestible energy MJ/kg	Weight/quart lb	Fibre %
Maize	14.7	1.7	2
Wheat	14.7	1.9	3
Barley	13.4	1.5	6
Rye	13.4	1.7	2
Oats	11.3	1.0	12

The most popular cereal for horses in the UK is undoubtedly oats. Perhaps because of this they may prove to be a relatively expensive source of energy. As can be seen from Table 20, they have the lowest digestible energy concentration and the lowest weight per volume of all the common cereals. These very facts also make oats the safest cereal for horses because owners are less likely to over-feed them. There is a further complication in that the quality of oats seems to vary more than that of the other cereals, with the result that the energy yield can vary from as low as 10MJ up to as high as 12.6MJ of digestible energy per 2.2lb (kg) of oats. Quality variations may also show in the amount of dust present in oats. It is important to realise that a horse should not be fed by giving X amount of oats for energy and Y amount of hay for protein. Each component of the ration will contribute to most of the various nutritional categories. So, although oats may have a lower energy content than corn (maize), they have a higher content of better quality protein than corn does. Crimping the oats can improve their energy availability by 7-10 per cent.

Corn (maize), which is extremely popular in certain countries such as the USA, has a higher digestible energy than oats and so needs more care in its feeding if problems are not to arise. Far from being the 'hot' food that some people consider it, corn will actually produce less heat than the conventional oats when the weights fed of the two are adjusted so that similar amounts of digestible energy are being fed. This is because the higher fibre content of oats can also be utilised to produce heat.

Barley has a digestible energy level somewhere in between that of oats and corn. It must be crimped or rolled before it is fed to horses. Steam-flaking barley merely produces the same effect as crimping or rolling, it does not make the cereal less heating. Other cereals, such as rye or wheat, can be used as energy sources for horses but, for a variety of reasons, care is necessary in their use.

Hay naturally has a much lower digestible energy concentration than cereals. Although legume hays (such as alfalfa, clover and bird's-foot trefoil) generally have higher levels of digestible energy, protein, calcium and vitamins than grass hays (such as fescue, timothy or blue-grass), you should remember that the quality of the individual hay you are buying is more important than the plants which it comprises. Legume hay, for instance, is more likely to become mouldy or dusty through incorrect storage than grass hay. To make good hay you must start off with the right ingredients. In deciding exactly when to make the hay, a balance must be struck between young plants which have a higher concentration of energy and older plants which have more fibre but which give a greater weight of end product per acre. Timothy, for instance, contains its highest protein levels (15 per cent) when still in the leaf stage, but has its highest energy levels when the flower heads first develop. Alfalfa also contains its highest protein levels (19 per cent) at the leaf stage, but has its highest energy levels when in early bud.

Fond though horses may be of sugar-lumps as a treat, it is unlikely that they will consume enough to make a significant contribution to their energy requirements in even the most indulgent household. Sugar-beet pulp has almost as high a concentration of digestible energy as an average sample of oats, giving 11MJ per 2.2lb (kg). It should never be fed just as it comes, however, because it can absorb liquid so rapidly that it swells enormously while passing down the oesophagus and becomes stuck there. Sugar-beet pulp should always be soaked in cold water for at least twelve hours, and nuts and pellets for twenty-four hours, before being fed, by which time it has already swollen up as much as it is going to do. This process naturally affects both its volume and its digestible energy per lb (kg) weight. In areas where it is readily available, sugar-beet pulp can be a very economical source of energy. Contrary to what one might think, cane molasses has a slightly lower digestible energy level than beet pulp (10MJ per 2.2lb (kg)). Demand for molasses for other purposes may well keep the price relatively high per unit of energy provided.

Feeding fat
The use of fat as a potential high source of energy to the horse has already been mentioned. Despite comments sometimes made in the popular equestrian press, horses will consume high amounts of fat without any digestive disturbances. The advantage of feeding fat is that on a weight basis it contains twice as much energy as carbohydrates, and therefore where the horse has to consume a large amount of feed to meet

its energy requirements, it is an extremely good source and reduces bulk in the digestive tract. In other words, it is a concentrated form of energy. The fat is added to the diet in the form of oil such as soya bean, or maize oil. Although these are not natural constituents normally, being only 1-2 per cent of the diet, it has been found that quantities up to 20 per cent of the diet can be well tolerated. As well as being a means of getting extra energy into animals with very high requirements, it has also been suggested – although good proof is lacking – that feeding fats helps adapt the muscle to use greater quantities of free fatty acids in place of glycogen during exercise. As described in an earlier chapter, this should prolong endurance times.

Feeding for proteins

Proteins, the building blocks of the body, are large complex molecules composed of up to twenty different amino acids. The amino acids are used to build and repair cells and tissues, to form enzymes, haemoglobin and plasma proteins; to form certain hormones and, under extreme circumstances, to provide energy. There are two groups of amino acids: those that are considered as essential and have to be provided in the diet, and those non-essential ones which can be produced by the body. Essential amino acids include lysine and methionine, and these are often included in supplements as many natural feeds are low in these amino acids. However, whether sufficient is added via supplementation is questionable.

As the body is continually breaking down muscle cells, etc, and replacing them with new ones, even mature horses need a certain amount of protein in their diet. Young growing animals naturally need even higher levels. When considering a horse's ration, the protein is usually measured as the percentage crude protein. It is possible to feed too much protein to a horse. If you do, the excess is broken down in its body. Part of the molecule will be used to provide energy and the nitrogen will be excreted in the urine. Because protein tends to be an expensive part of the ration, and because the horse has to use energy to break down and remove this excess protein, it is very uneconomical to feed too much protein. Feeding too much protein to young growing horses has also been claimed by some to cause crooked legs and other deformities. If this occurs it may be due to the fact that many protein sources are also good sources of minerals such as calcium and phosphorus. So, although the feeding of these protein-rich feedstuffs can all too readily cause a mineral imbalance, this is because they supply the minerals in the wrong proportions rather than because of any other reason. There is some evidence that high-protein levels can have a deleterious effect on a horse's performance.

Table 21   The dietary protein requirements of the horse

Type of Horse	Protein requirement as percentage of food
Mature working horse	7.7
Mare in late pregnancy	10.0
Mare in early lactation	12.5
Six month foal	14.5
Yearling	12.0
Two-year-old	9.0

When considering how much protein should be fed, it has been estimated that the requirements can vary from 7.7 per cent to 16 per cent of the diet on a dry-matter basis (Table 21). For a long time it has been claimed that exercise greatly increases the amount of protein that should be fed. This claim has developed both from the idea that with exercise extra protein is required for building muscle bulk and also to prevent the breakdown of muscle during exercise. One of the greatest influences for the trend for high protein diets has been the image of enormous steak dinners being consumed by human athletes, most notably weight-lifters. These suggestions for high protein has lead to the formulation of horse diets containing around 20 per cent crude protein. In reality the latest evidence indicates that such diets are unnecessary, with even some indications that they may be undesirable.

Although there is an increased daily requirement for protein with exercise the general consensus of equine nutritionists is that these increases are met by the overall increase in ration fed to the horse to meet its energy requirements. For example, if a horse at rest was eating 8.5kg of feed containing 7.7 per cent crude protein, he would receive 655g of protein daily. When working he may eat 15.5kg of feed and obtain 1194g daily. The increased requirement comes about through nitrogen loss in sweat and some increase in muscle mass. Requirements for the latter will obviously be greater in two- and three-year-olds than mature horses, and also in the early stages of a training programme.

Therefore, there should be no necessity to exceed 8 per cent protein in the diet. A recent study concludes that even 5.5 per cent is sufficient. As most reasonable hays contain at least 7 per cent protein, with oats and barley 11 to 14 per cent, and corn 9.6 per cent, there is, therefore, no place for protein supplementation. As already discussed there may be a point in supplementing with certain amino acids; however, further work in this area is required to ascertain the correct amounts.

Grazing, especially if it has a high clover content, may contain as much as 20 per cent protein on a dry-matter basis. Unfortunately, quality and digestibility appear to be linked. Pastures with a high leaf content have a high digestibility level, whereas those with a higher stem content are less digestible but also of lower protein quality. A ration which is balanced to allow for poor quality protein must also be increased to cater for the fact that the protein will not be digested as efficiently.

Hay is a significant, although very variable (2-18 per cent dry matter), source of protein. Legume hay may cause horses to urinate more than usual because it provides too much protein for the mature animal and the excess nitrogen which is left behind when this has been broken down has to be excreted by the urine. Top quality alfalfa hays are therefore best fed to young growing horses or mares with a foal at foot (not the classes of animal that usually get the pick of the hay crops) so that their high-protein content is not wasted. It must always be remembered that the nutritional quality of hay is extremely variable, especially in temperate climates. A recent survey in the UK found that digestible energy levels varied from 5.7 to 10.5MJ per 2.2lb (kg). One can contemplate hay providing an athletic horse with its maintenance requirements for energy and protein, but only as long as it did not stride out of the stable. The requirements for even light work must come from elsewhere. The other vegetable sources of good quality protein will vary, depending on your geographical location. Soya-bean meal, for example, is a very good and economical protein source in the USA (Table 22), but much less so in western Europe where it has to be imported. Animal proteins, such as milk powder, are very high-quality protein sources, but tend to be relatively expensive.

Table 22   Vegetable sources of protein

Feed Source	Protein %	Quality (percentage of lysine)
Alfalfa Hay	14	5.6
Brewers Grains	27	3.3
Fish Meal	72	7.9
Linseed Meal	33	3.6
Skimmed Milk Powder	33	7.8
Soya-bean Meal	45	6.7

Ever since experiments at the Irish National Stud in the 1970s showed that silage could be safely fed to horses, small numbers of owners have been doing so. The advent of polythene-packed big bale silage seemed to offer advantages of storage, standardisation of quality, etc. Unfortunately, a number of horses eating this roughage have died as a result of botulism (a rapidly fatal disease caused by a member of the Clostridial family of bacteria). When owners wish to continue to use big bale silage on economic grounds, they should check that a preservative was used and inspect every bale to make sure that the polythene has not been punctured. Any bales where the pH of the fluid in the silage is significantly higher than 4.5 should be immediately discarded.

Compound feeds

Because of the difficulties in feeding balanced diets, the problems in obtaining grains and hay of uniform consistency and also costs, the popularity of coarse mixes, cube or pelleted feeds has increased markedly over the last twenty years, although such feeds were introduced as early as 1917. These rations have the advantage in that their composition is always uniform, and this gives the horse owner increased confidence that the correct quantities of protein, etc are fed. These preparations also have less dust, require less storage space and are generally less wasteful. Also, savings are made in the time taken for feeding as formulation of rations is not required. As shown in Table 23, different formulations of these pelleted feeds are available and this again makes it easier to adjust the diet according to how hard the horse is working. For the endurance horse, there are preparations available incorporating a high percentage of fat (oil). Generally, pelleted feeds are fed in conjunction with hay in order to provide the bulk for the large intestine to function correctly. The eating of hay also reduces boredom and the development of undesirable vices such as crib-biting and the eating of its own droppings. In deciding which pelleted feed to use, not only does the composition with respect to digestible energy and protein have to be considered, but also its palatability. It is well known that some horses can be fussy eaters, and on occasions these feeds may not be immediately acceptable. This should be borne in mind when changing from the preparation of one manufacturer to another. In any case, any change to a high-energy pelleted feed should be done gradually to avoid any digestive disturbances leading to colic.

Table 23 Major nutrients in different compound feeds of one manufacturer to be fed for different levels of activity

		Complete* Cubes	Horse and Pony Cubes	Special Event Cubes	Racehorse Cubes
Crude protein	%	10	10.5	10.5	14.0
Fibre	%	20	14.0	14.5	9.5
Oil	%	2.5	2.5	2.5	3.25
Ash	%	8.5	10.3	9.5	7.50
Approximate digestible energy (MJ/kg dm)		9.6	10.1	10.7	13.4

*This feed has a higher proportion of fibre and can be fed without hay. All other feeds require hay to be fed as well.

Supplements

Many horse owners are quite happy to leave the question of providing a ration balanced for energy and protein to the manufacturers of commercial nuts and rations. However, curiously enough, they will, at the same time, insist that they know better than the experts when it comes to providing the correct minerals, vitamins and other substances in the form of supplements. Some owners/trainers will even use more than one of these preparations containing the same substances. This is in addition to a so-called balanced diet. Obviously, supplements are also extensively used to complement diets prepared by the trainer and here certain ones may be essential. The term supplement refers to all the additional preparations that may be added to the horse's normal feed. The various additives used in supplements can be divided into the following categories:

1 Minerals, trace elements, electrolytes.
2 Vitamins.
3 Bacterial cultures and other compounds to improve digestibility.
4 Miscellaneous, including such substances as ginseng, pangamic acid, etc, which may or may not be allowed under the rules of racing for that country.

An enormous number of single or multi-substance supplements are marketed, with their prices often being far in excess of what their individual substances cost (Fig 41). These supplements may be fed in order to correct dietary imbalances either real or imaginary, to improve questionably digestibility or just in response to usually unsubstantiated claims that a certain substance may give the horse that extra performance advantage. Often, the introduction of such substances to equine supplements closely follows their 'in vogue' use in man. Even if a substance, eg electrolytes, may be beneficial, often little attention is given by manufacturers to whether the correct amount is added, the quantity used being dictated by economic rather than efficacy considerations. It is not unknown that a compound may be added to a supplement so that enquiries by a trainer on its presence can be answered positively, despite it being in inadequate amounts. An example of this will be illustrated at the end of this chapter.

Despite being critical of supplements so far, there is undoubtedly a place for some, and in deciding which ones, perhaps the following points should be considered:

1 Under normal nutritional programmes, is a deficiency in this substance likely to occur, and are requirements increased by hard work?
2 Will the substance have a synergistic, additive, or antagonistic effect with other substances?
3 What are the chances of toxicity? This is especially important when trace elements are administered.
4 What is the cost?

In the absence of any likelihood of toxicity occurring, it is more often cost that is the determining factor, especially when inconclusive evidence of a compound's efficacy is available. It should be pointed out that often it is very difficult to prove a substance's usefulness in improving performance. It is obvious that the cost-effectiveness will vary between different racing stables, or even eventers. In stables where hundreds of thousands of pounds are spent on each animal, there can be little argument against using supplements which may only add a few pounds to the week's training costs in the slight hope that they may be of use or correct an imbalance in only one of fifty horses, without any deleterious effects in the other animals. However, in many stables where economics are crucial, the use of dubious supplements has to be more closely examined. Overall, for the average competition horse the position on the use of supplements has little changed from a comment passed in 1906, 'These feeds are too expensive'. If your animals are in good health, they need no tonic feeds. If they are sick, it is cheaper to consult a veterinarian!

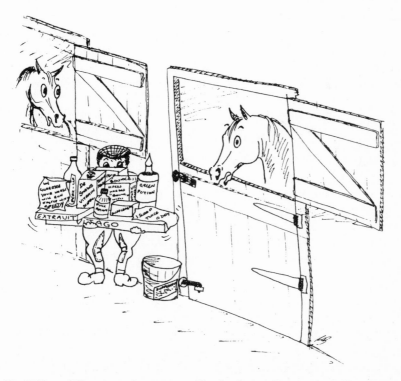

Fig 41 Many different supplements are offered to horses (drawing by J. Cornelius)

Minerals and trace elements

The role and necessity for supplementation with certain minerals has already been discussed in earlier chapters. However, some of the problems in feeding extra minerals will be described here. The tendency is for people to know merely that certain minerals, for example, are essential and they then just feed extra of these minerals. It is actually much more complicated than that because the requirements and the absorption of many minerals are inter-related. If we take calcium as an example, because it is a mineral which everyone is aware of, the levels of calcium in a horse's diet will markedly affect how much phosphorus, magnesium, zinc and copper are absorbed from that same diet. That is not the end of the problem, however, because the very levels of phosphorus, magnesium or iron in the diet can of themselves influence absorption of calcium! It is not just the minerals which can affect the absorption of other minerals either. Some proteins, carbohydrates, fats and vitamins can also alter calcium availability one way or another. Nor is it sufficient to feed merely high levels of a deficient mineral in the diet. Feeding a very high level of calcium does not produce any marked effect on the levels of calcium in the horse's blood because the bone of the skeleton acts as a reservoir which keeps the blood levels constant. It follows that measuring the blood levels of the mineral calcium will not be much help in diagnosing bone problems due to mineral deficiency, because blood levels do not reflect bone levels. In fact, bone levels may be lowered even further simply to maintain blood levels at a constant level.

Because their presence in feeds and their absorption are closely linked, it is customary to consider calcium and phosphorus together. They are far and away the commonest minerals in the horse's body. More than 99 per cent of the calcium and 80 per cent of the phosphorus are in the bones as a chemical called hydroxyapatite. This does not contain equal amounts of the two minerals – the calcium : phosphorus ratio is about 2:1. Despite the fact that such a high proportion of these minerals is bound up in the bone forming the skeleton, they do have other, just as vital, functions. Calcium is involved in blood clotting, muscle contraction and the transmission of nerve impulses. Phosphorus is a vital component of many of the essential chemicals in the body, especially some of the enzymes, the substances which help to change one chemical into another inside the cells. It has already been mentioned that the skeleton acts as a reservoir of calcium. It is important to point out that calcium is not actually taken out of the skeleton. What happens is that bones, far from being inert, are constantly forming new bone crystals and destroying others. Indeed, we rely on this for fracture repair, etc. When calcium needs to be taken from storage in the skeleton, what happens is that the normal breakdown of hydroxyapatite goes on but much less new apatite is formed. There is then much less of this crystal in the bone. The bone is then less dense and less able to withstand stress. A young horse which is short of calcium will still grow in height. The bones will grow longer but will be less dense and more liable to injury. Table 24 shows the calcium and phosphorus requirements of horses, based on a 1,100lb (500kg) horse. Table 25 shows how these requirements can be met using 'crude' chemicals rather than packaged supplements. Note that the cheapest way to add calcium to the diet is to feed some ground limestone.

Table 24   Calcium and phosphorus requirements of the horse

| | Daily requirements | |
	Calcium	Phosphorus
Foal	33g	20g
Yearling	31g	22g
Two-year-old	25g	17g
Mare in late pregnancy	50g	34g
Mature horse, maintenance only	23g	14g

Table 25   Calcium and phosphorus levels in horse feeds

	Gm of Calcium per 30g	Gm of Phos per 30g	% Calcium absorbed	% Phos absorbed
Bonemeal	9	4	71	46
Monosodium Phosphate	0	7	–	47
Limestone	10	0	67	–
Maize	1.5	18	–	38
Wheat Bran	0.04	0.34	–	34
Timothy Hay	0.12	0.06	70	42
Alfalfa	0.39	0.08	77	38

As described in Chapter 7 when we look at the question of salt supplements for the horse, it should be appreciated that its normal diet is high in potassium and low in sodium. This is the opposite of the situation in man. So, if anything causes a loss of sodium, it is possible for a deficiency to occur. This may be the situation when prolonged sweating occurs, because horse sweat has a high concentration of sodium and potassium. The potassium lost in this way will generally be replaced from the diet, but the sodium may not be. It is therefore recommended that where prolonged or pronounced sweating occurs due to exercise or hot, humid conditions, a salt-lick or other extra salt should be given. Although there are numerous electrolyte preparations available, the cheapest way of doing this is by using table salt (about 2oz (60g) per day per horse). Bicarbonate is often given to horses shortly prior to racing. The idea behind this is to improve the buffering capacity of the blood. It is unlikely that the buffering capacity of muscle itself is increased, but the affect on the blood may speed up removal of intramuscular lactate and so delay the damaging effects of lactate accumulation.

Iron is another mineral which everyone has heard of, and is one which everyone wants to supplement. It is a most important part of the haemoglobin molecule which carries oxygen around in the red blood cells. It is also a very important constituent of myoglobin in muscles. So the horse certainly needs some iron in its diet. Luckily, a diet which is of a reasonable quality will provide the forty parts per million that the mature horse needs. As a further help in this direction, the body is extremely careful about wasting iron. Very little iron is ever excreted from the body, although some is lost in sweat; it is reabsorbed and used again. Where so many well-meaning horse owners go wrong is to assume that because a horse needs a certain amount of iron to keep up its haemoglobin levels, feeding extra iron will automatically raise these levels. This is not the case; iron is not the limiting factor in deciding whether a horse has low levels of haemoglobin. Nor, despite some of the advertising for so-called 'haematinics', or blood tonics, does giving iron stimulate the manufacture of more red blood cells. When, of course, a horse is diagnosed as suffering from anaemia, an iron tonic may cure the problem. The important thing in such cases is that once the problem has been diagnosed the owner should change all sort of things besides the iron supplement. If you take a horse out of the field and do nothing except give it extra iron in its food, you will not produce a single extra red blood cell or a single extra gram of haemoglobin.

One trace element whose importance is difficult to evaluate in the athletic horse is selenium. This element is a vital part of an enzyme called glutathione peroxidase which, in association with vitamin E, is responsible for the mopping up of substances referred to as free radicals. These radicals are substances that are produced under certain circumstances and can be very destructive to the cell unless rapidly removed. Whether there is an increased production of these radicals with exercise is largely unknown. However, because of this possibility and diets generally being low in both selenium and vitamin E, most manufactured diets have extra amounts of these substances added, and trainers use supplements containing these if mixing their own rations. Normally, a very minute amount, ie 1mg per day of selenium is given in a supplement. It should be appreciated that excess can be toxic. Recent studies by one of the authors indicates that at least in racehorses, there is no necessity for selenium supplementation even if diets are below normally accepted levels. It has been found that a deficiency of either selenium or vitamin

E can cause muscle disease in certain species and in young horses. From these findings it has been suggested that a deficiency of either of these may also play a role in causing exertional rhabdomyolysis (ie tying-up, azoturia or set fast) and muscular weakness. Therefore, some veterinary surgeons treat the condition by giving extra selenium and/or vitamin E. However, recent work does not support the idea of tying-up being due to low levels of these substances in the muscle.

Vitamins
The whole field of vitamin supplements for performance is a real minefield. This is also true in the human world, where our packets of breakfast cereals tell us that if we eat four bowlsful we will have consumed our full day's requirements of most of the important vitamins. This is no great advantage, though, because we would probably eat more than adequate amounts in other meals. Athletes and health-food fanatics have been known to consume megadoses of vitamins, to the benefit of the manufacturer rather than themselves. This is not the place for a detailed look at the role of every vitamin in the horse, but rather we shall look at the vitamins which might be in short supply in the horse under the stress of competition. The role of each vitamin is summarised in Table 26.

Vitamin A is important for vision and bone growth. It also has a more widespread role in the formation of epithelial cells, the cells which form the surface or lining of the skin, respiratory system, etc. The horse obtains most of its vitamin A from a substance called carotene which it absorbs and stores in the liver until needed. Green feeds contain good levels of carotene, but much of this is destroyed during the drying which converts the grass, etc to hay. The activity of vitamin A supplements can also be destroyed by poor storage. Horses in training which have not had regular access to grazing for several months should have some vitamin A supplementation. Although there is little information on the daily requirements of vitamin A for a working horse, it appears that 50,000iu should be given as a supplement.

The B-group vitamin, thiamine, (vit B_1) has an important role in energy production inside the individual cells. Without it pyruvic acid and lactic acid cannot be broken down. This means both that toxic levels of these acids may accumulate and also that blood glucose levels will drop. Horses in strong work may well benefit from extra thiamine, despite the fact that cereals have good levels of the vitamin. Horse owners should be aware that horses do not require any vitamin B_{12} (cyanocobolamin) supplement at all. Attempts to produce any symptoms of vitamin B_{12} deficiency in horses have all failed. Indeed, so

Table 26   The function and source of vitamins in the horse

Vitamin	Function	Natural Source
1 FAT-SOLUBLE		
A	Vision, integrity of skin and mucous membranes, connective tissue, resistance to infection	Green forage
D	Bone growth and strength by influencing mineralisation of bone, regulation of calcium and phosphorus	Sunlight; sun-cured hay
E	As an antioxidant to prevent breakdown of other vitamins and fats	Grains
K	Manufacture of several factors required in blood clotting	High in plants, synthesised in large intestine
2 WATER-SOLUBLE		
B_1 (thiamine)	Involved in carbohydrate metabolism	Leafy plants, sun-cured hay, grains
B_2 (riboflavin)	Energy metabolism	High in yeasts, in hay, low in grain
B_3 (niacin, nicotinic acid)	Energy metabolism, fatty acid synthesis	In feeds, or produced from tryptophan in the body
B_6 (pyridoxine)	Protein metabolism, production of energy	In grass
B_{12} (cyanocobolamin)	Formation of red blood cells	Produced by bacteria in large intestine
Folic acid	Formation of red blood cells	In green forage, produced by bacteria in large intestine
Pantothenic acid	Aerobic metabolism	In most feeds
Biotin	Protein and energy metabolism, hoof keratinisation	
Vitamin C	Formation of collagen, removal of free radicals; ? resistance to infection	Produced by the body

much of this vitamin is manufactured inside the horse that even if you feed it none at all, there will still be large amounts discarded into the faeces. Conversely, feeding extra vitamin B_{12} to horses has not been shown to increase either the number of red blood cells they possess or the amount of haemoglobin which those cells are carrying. There is some evidence that folic acid does affect the manufacture of red blood cells. Because this vitamin is normally found in good quality grazing, especially that with a high legume content, horses which are permanently stabled can become deficient. These horses then show rather low red blood cell counts, ie they are anaemic. Giving a folic acid supplement to these horses is the only situation where it has been scientifically proved that a supplement has caused the horse to make more blood cells. Feeding good quality legume hay to horses which are stabled all the time for training may help to maintain folic acid levels (most of the vitamin is destroyed during the drying of the hay-making process), but it may be advisable to give a folic acid supplement to be on the safe side. Because the vitamin is so poorly absorbed from such supplements, very high levels are needed, far higher than those usually contained in commercial supplements.

Another vitamin where oral administration can be difficult but where recent evidence suggests it may be worthwhile is ascorbic acid, or vitamin C. Like most animals, but unlike man, the horse can produce its own ascorbic acid. Blood levels of ascorbic acid have, however, been found to be reduced under conditions of stress, in horses suffering from respiratory virus problems, and in those suffering from what is called the 'loss of performance syndrome'. The vitamin is thought to be involved in certain immune responses to viruses, etc and to affect the manufacture of natural corticosteroids among other functions. Originally, it was thought that giving ascorbic acid by mouth was a waste of time because it was not absorbed. This turns out not to be the case. Giving 20g per day of ascorbic acid has now been shown to raise the plasma levels in treated horses. Studies in man have shown no evidence that administering high doses of ascorbic acid to normal healthy people improves performance, but perhaps, as has been suggested for many years, administration may help to resist infectious diseases during times of increased stress. It is not included in pelleted or cube feeds owing to the instability of vitamin C.

The important role of vitamin E has already been discussed in conjunction with selenium. This vitamin is usually added to feeds or given as a supplement because in hay-making and the milling of seeds, much of the naturally occurring vitamin E is destroyed. Often, very large amounts of vitamin E are given as toxicity has not been seen and is unlikely. However, from a recent report from Sweden in Standardbreds it appears that the optimum amount per day was between 600-1,800iu or mg of di-alpha-toco-pheryl-acetate (a form of vitamin E). It was also found that it is better to give this vitamin on a daily basis, rather than larger doses less frequently. Higher levels of vitamin E may be required if extra fat or propionate-treated hay is fed.

Recently, a few supplement manufacturers have promoted the use of the vitamin biotin as an aid to healthy strong horn growth. Within a very short time, most of the vitamin supplements contained the vitamin and made similar claims. The scientific basis for these claims in the horse is very scanty. Before introducing a biotin supplement specifically to improve the quality of the horn in your horse's feet, it is important to remember that it will be several months before any vitamin-influenced horm comes into wear along the hoof wall. It may also be true that a good farrier can do more for a horse's feet than a vitamin supplement.

Evaluation of a supplement

As has already been mentioned, because of the lack of adequate information in many instances, it can be very difficult to decide whether certain constituents and the amounts used are correct. However, as will now be shown, many supplements can be evaluated and shown to be essentially worthless. In the writers' opinion, such an example of an available electrolyte preparation is documented with explanations below.

Table 27   Example of an electrolyte and glucose preparation commercially available, but of little benefit

A total of 40g, given once per day, is broken down as follows:

	Amount
Sodium chloride	2.6g
Potassium chloride	1.7g
Magnesium sulphate	0.2g
Sodium hydrogen phosphate	0.15g
Sodium citrate	0.16g
Sodium phosphate	0.65g
Ascorbic acid	0.45g
Glucose	20.2g
Sucrose	9.0g
Yeast torula	4.5g

Total sodium	= approximately 1.3g
Total potassium	= approximately 0.9g

Energy from glucose + sucrose = approximately 0.5MJ, an amount that will sustain just over one minute of exercise at 50 per cent VO_2 max ie at a medium trot, if an equal amount of fat is also used.

10 · Drugs: Their Use and Abuse

Doping

Chemical compounds which, when administered, elicit a response within the body are considered as drugs. Although the word drug conjures up in many minds the detrimental use of a compound, it must be remembered that, in the vast majority of instances, such compounds are used for their beneficial effect in treating injuries and disease. The beneficial effects are those related to therapy, whether for physical or mental disorders. The detrimental effects are generally considered when normally safe compounds are used either in abnormally high amounts or specifically to produce various actions on the central nervous system leading to alterations in normal behavioural patterns.

The words dope and doping have been used to refer to the illicit administration of compounds to alter performance, ie enhance or impair. The word dope is considered to be of recent origin and derived from the Dutch word *dope,* which is the name of a type of brandy made from grape skins in South Africa. A local hard liquor of this was used by the Kaffirs as a stimulant. However, in the horse doping has to be considered in a wider context, as it should also include their possible use in masking abnormalities at sales and therefore incorrectly influencing a prospective buyer. For example, anti-inflammatory agents or analgesic drugs have been used to hide lamenesses, or mild tranquillisers to make intractable horses appear placid. In young animals anabolic steroids have been used to increase muscle bulk and thus appearance. Once the animal is purchased and the anabolic steroid is removed, weight is then lost.

Attempts to alter performance by the ingestion of various compounds is as old as competitions involving man, with references dating back to ancient Greece and Rome, although, interestingly, the first proven case of doping was in 1910 on a saliva test taken from a horse. In the early days, doping was confined to the use of compounds that were extracts of various parts of plants, but today it has evolved to such a degree that compounds are being specifically manufactured that have no therapeutic usefulness, as well as those that have a therapeutic application. Today's drugs are not only given orally but also by injection into tissues or directly into the blood in order to enhance or speed up the action of the compound. Not only are single compounds used, but often cocktail-mixtures containing a variety of compounds with differing actions. In attempts to try to avoid detection in dope tests, other drugs are used to try to dilute and/or mask their presence. It has even been said that in some countries the desire to use drugs to obtain unfair advantages has led to additional competition between the ingenuity of chemists to manufacture new compounds of ever-increasing specificity and potency and on the other side, the drug analysts' ability to develop more and more sophisticated techniques to detect the newer compounds at the very low dose rates used.

Regulations on drug use before competition

The administration of compounds to influence performance is widely classed as doping, and as such is considered an illegal activity undertaken by subterfuge, although on occasions it occurs accidentally or through ignorance. However, what actually constitutes a doping agent not only takes into consideration the effects they may have on performance, but also whether they may have short- or long-term risks to the health of the individual. For example, the use of amphetamines has led to the death of a number of athletes owing to their inability to perceive fatigue, while anabolic steroids may have long-term deleterious effects by causing damage to certain tissues, eg the liver. The International Olympic Committee has listed substances that are illegal for use in Olympic competition. In addition, international and national organisers of different sporting disciplines are now devising their own regulations and testing procedures to counteract criticisms on the abuse of drugs in sport.

In the equestrian and racing world, differing regulations exist on the use of drugs in horses. At one extreme is the rule presently in force in the UK and a number of other countries with respect to Thoroughbred racing. This rule indicates that, at the time of running, the horse is now allowed to show the presence of *any* quantity of *any* substance in its tissues, body fluids or excreta, which is either prohibited, or the origin of which cannot be traced to normal and ordinary feeding and which could, by its nature, affect the racing performance of the horse. This has lead to the guideline for veterinarians to avoid giving any drug, therapeutic or otherwise, within eight days of racing, and for some drug preparations, even longer. Therefore, even drugs such as antibiotics, which could have no effect on performance, are excluded from use. However, it does not exclude supplementation with high doses of vitamins, electrolytes and trace elements. An advantage of such an all-encompassing rule is that there is no requirement for the regulatory body to provide evidence as to whether a blood or urine level of a drug indicates that the dose administered was likely to influence performance. This is important because of the near impossibility of obtaining such information, as well as deciding whether a drug truly improves performance in a normal healthy horse. For example, if a stimulant can improve performance by 1 per cent, this can mean the difference between winning or finishing last. However, such small differences can be very difficult to detect in experimental tests.

List of prohibited substances under rules of the Jockey Club (Great Britain)
Drugs acting on the central nervous system
Drugs acting on the automatic nervous system
Drugs acting on the cardiovascular system
Drugs affecting the gastro-intestinal function
Drugs affecting the immune system and its response

Antibiotics, synthetic anti-bacterial and anti-viral drugs
Antihistamines
Anti-malarials and anti-parasitic agents
Anti-pyretics, analgesic and anti-inflammatory drugs
Diuretics
Local anaesthetics
Muscle relaxants
Respiratory stimulants
Sex hormones, anabolic agents and corticosteroids
Endocrine secretions and their synthetic counterparts
Substances affecting blood coagulation
Cytotoxic substances

In other countries, more lenient rules are in existence. For example, in Japan only drugs named in a list are illegal which means that it is possible to always remain one step ahead of the analysts and racing authorities. Within the USA, regulations vary widely between different states and racing authorities. In most states, there are rules which allow the use of therapeutic agents as well as some, such as anti-inflammatory drugs, which can influence performance. In those instances there is a distinction between illegal medication constituting doping and legally controlled or permissive medication where drugs can be legitimately administered for therapeutic purposes on or near to race days. The rules governing controlled medications vary widely, especially with respect to the amount of drug that can be used, and the minimum time between administration and racing. Where permissive or controlled medication is allowed, rules are usually set down for the use of the anti-inflammatory agent phenylbutazone (bute) and the diuretic frusemide (Lasix). In the international controlling body of equestrian events, the FEI enforces similar rules to those operating for racing in the United Kingdom, with the exception of phenylbutazone. The use of this drug is allowed as long as plasma concentrations of phenylbutazone and an active metabolite, oxyphenbutazone, do not exceed 5 iug/ml at the time of sampling.

However, when considering what regulations are used, their enforcement can only be as good as the expertise of the analytical laboratories examining the samples. In trying to detect the presence of illegal compounds, fluids from the body are examined. Generally, this fluid is urine which is collected following competition, while in some circumstances, it can also be blood or saliva, although the latter has largely fallen into disuse. In addition to the collection of post-race samples, some jurisdictions, eg in Hong Kong, also resort to the collection of pre-race samples. These are analysed prior to racing and any horses showing suspicions of doping are not permitted to run. The advantage of this system is that betting coups due to doping can be averted, as well as just fining the owner/trainer of the offending animal. Again, in some jurisdictions all animals are tested, but in others, because of the expense of this testing, examination is restricted to place getters, horses performing below expectations and a random selection. Once the samples are within the analyst's laboratory, various tests, often requiring very expensive equipment, are carried out. Once a positive sample is detected, its presence has to be generally confirmed using other methods before action is taken. For the reader who is interested in a detailed account of the history of horserace doping, the drugs used and detection methods, the excellent book on this subject, *Drugs and the Performance Horse,* by Professor Tom Tobin and published by Charles C. Thomas, Illinois (1981), should be read.

In trying to consider rationally how drugs may influence performance and whether they may be truly considered as doping agents, we must consider that the drugs can be classified into various categories which are tabulated below. From these categories we can see that drugs can be considered as those which are obviously doping agents, ie stimulants and depressants, and those where there may be some justification for their use.

1 Drugs that impair performance

a) Depressants. Various types of tranquillisers and sedatives have been used. These are usually administered as an 'outside job'.

b) Drugs that may inhibit the normal metabolic response to exercise, eg B-adrenergic blocking agents. These are used frequently in human medicine for the prevention of hypertension and cardiac conditions.

2 Drugs that improve performance

a) Stimulants. These are usually short-acting and are given prior to the competition. They include such compounds as amphetamines, cocaine and narcotics.

b) Drugs that restore normal performance, ie they are used to help overcome debilitating conditions that do not allow horses to perform to their full potential. In this category are anti-inflammatory drugs, eg phenylbutazone and corticosteroids, analgesics and local anaesthetics for removing pain and antibiotics, etc in the treatment of infection. The use of frusemide to alleviate exercise-induced pulmonary haemorrhage.

c) Training aids to help prevent the onset of fatigue can be given for a prolonged period, eg anabolic steroids, or prior to competition, eg bicarbonate, pangamic acid.

Whether drugs that restore normal performance should be permitted is debatable, and the pros and cons are considered shortly. The greyest area is whether drugs that improve performance by aiding in a higher level of fitness or the supply of energy at the level of muscle fibres should be permitted. When considering improvement in performance, this may be brought about either by increasing speed or by improving agility to aid co-ordination, or a combination of the two.

In considering the attempts to dope horses, figures are difficult to obtain as they are dependent on the detection of the drug or obvious clinical signs of medication. However, it does appear that in countries where a strict control is kept, very few incidences are reported. For example, in the UK over the past ten years, there have been only relatively few instances of positive results, and in the vast majority these have been accidental. The greatest number of positives were due to the formation of a compound called theobromine in the horse from caffeine, a normal constituent of some beverages such as tea and coffee. This compound is also found in many plants and therefore occasionally is incorporated into pelleted horse feeds when they are compounded. Because of these risks some feed manufacturers in the UK have special process lines to try to minimise the risk of contamination from feeds containing theobromine and that may be used in the pelleting of feeds for other species, eg cattle. On the other hand, in countries where controls are limited, it appears that drugs are used on a wider scale. It should also be stressed that attempts at doping are not restricted to racing, but are evident at all levels in which one competitor is trying to gain an advantage over another.

The use of different categories of compounds will now be considered.

Depressants and stimulants

The main function of the nervous system is communication, allowing co-ordination of responses between different organs in the body. Consequently, any compound affecting the central nervous system (CNS) may exert widespread physiological and psychological responses. These can be either of a stimulant or depressant nature, with some drugs exerting a stimulant effect at low doses and a depressant at higher doses. A number of classifications have been developed to categorise CNS drugs dependent upon their physiological and/or psychological actions. To describe the basic action of these compounds, terms used such as analgesic, hypnotic, sedative, tranquilliser, anti-depressant, narcotic, sympathomimetic, and hallucinogenic have been used. However, in a simplified manner they can be classed as either depressants or stimulants.

These drugs can exert their effects by the actions at the junctions between nerve cells at the various parts of the central nervous system, ie the brain and spinal cord. Normally, communication between nerve cells occurs by the passage of a chemical compound referred to as a neurotransmitter. This is released from one cell, then diffusion takes place across a very narrow gap to act on receptors located on another cell. Drugs may inhibit or accelerate production of the neurotransmitter, modify its rate of disappearance or affect its interaction with its receptors. How some drugs act in this manner is known, with the action of many being unknown, although the unravelling of the effects of many is progressing rapidly. For example, it has been discovered recently that morphine and many other narcotics exert their effects by mimicking the actions of a group of naturally occurring compounds referred to as endorphins or enkephalins.

Depressants

Until the 1950s only a few drugs were available to calm a nervous horse or, in higher doses, to depress the system to such an extent as to impair performance. The first drugs were chloral hydrate and barbiturates which were mainly employed as anaesthetics. However, since then drugs have been developed that are used for tranquillisation to permit easier treatment by veterinarians of intractable or nervous horses. These drugs have also been used in educating horses to do certain tasks they may at first feel anxious about, eg entering starting gates. These drugs essentially exert an action on the CNS which makes the animal less responsive to its surroundings. However, they also exert effects on other tissues. There are a number of drugs within the category of tranquillisers and commonly used ones include acetylpromazine (colloquially known as Ace), chlorpromazine (Largactil, a compound used infrequently in horses by veterinarians, but used widely in man – prospective dopers have easy access to it), and reserpine. Reserpine is a drug that has quite a prolonged effect, while the others are much shorter acting. In investigations on the effects of these tranquillisers on performance, it has been found that a reduction in running speed and co-ordination occurs if a sufficient dose is used. In addition, the minor tranquillisers, such as diazepam (Valium^R) and chlordiazepoxide (Librium^R), have been employed, although no reports are available on what effects they have on the horse.

In addition to those depressant drugs that act on the CNS, there is another group which can impair the normal metabolic and physiological response to exercise. Nature has evolved the compound adrenalin, which is released during times of danger to the animal. It has been referred to as the fright flight or fight hormone, as it allows most of the adjustments referred to in previous chapters, ie, increase in heart rate, increased respiration, increase in glucose and free fatty acids in the blood. Recently, a group of drugs has been manufactured that can block some of the actions of adrenalin and have found use in man in the treatment of hypertension and cardiac diseases. These compounds are referred to as B-adrenergic blocking drugs. They have been found to reduce performance capacity in both the horse and man. In addition, because of their reducing heart-rate elevations they have been employed by athletes involved in shooting disciplines and also in dressage horses to improve steadiness.

Stimulants
In general, this group of drugs increase the excitability of the nerve cells in the CNS, facilitating the processes of both sensory input and motor output. Stimulants used in horses can be grouped into several classes: amphetamines and similar agents; cocaine; caffeine and other xanthines; narcotics; psychotomimetics; miscellaneous.

Amphetamines amphetamine, methylamphetamine, methylphenidate (Ritalin), ephedrine) In human athletes, and probably also in the horse, this has been one of the most frequently used of the illegal drugs. These drugs act by mimicking the action of nor-adrenalin (nor epinephrine) within the CNS. Their effect is to influence the CNS to produce subjective or objective mental and physical changes which may increase performance capacity. They may have physiological effects such as increasing cardiac output, increasing respiratory rate, increasing oxygen uptake, increased blood flow to muscle and increased cerebral activity. Biochemically, they can increase the delivery of glucose and free fatty acids to muscle. In other words, they are able to prime the body for increased energy expenditure. However, whether this does result in an innate improvement in speed is controversial, with both improvements and no difference being reported in scientific literature. In the horse, improvements in running speed have been described. Of less controversy is their ability to prolong performance capacity by delaying the sense of fatigue, ie it removes some inhibitory influences. For this purpose, it found widespread use in soldiers in World War II. This delaying of fatigue means that the early warning signs that the body's capacity is being exceeded are missed and if exercise is prolonged for too long, deleterious effects can result. There have been a number of instances in man where athletes competing under the influence of amphetamines have driven themselves to death.

Cocaine   This is an alkaloid derived from plants, and has been used for centuries by natives in Peru and Bolivia where leaves were chewed for its stimulant activity. As well as having stimulant actions on the CNS, it also has a local anaesthetic effect. It was the first local anaesthetic used in medicine. Today, procaine and lignocaine (Xylocaine) are much more commonly used. An extract from coca leaves was utilised in numerous commercial preparations including Coca-Cola during the nineteenth century.

Its action is claimed to be through its effect on allowing nor-adrenalin to accumulate within certain areas of the brain. In man and animals it causes an increased restlessness, seen in animals as increased movement. Its duration of activity is much shorter than the amphetamines. It is also claimed that it removes the sensation of fatigue. However, in both man and horse, there are few reports on its effectiveness. The 1980s has seen an enormous increase in the illegal use of this drug in all classes of society, including sportsmen. The ease of its detection in drugs-testing procedures makes its illegal use unlikely in racehorses, and over the years very few positive cases have been reported.

Caffeine and other xanthines   Caffeine and theobromine belong to a group of compounds which are referred to as xanthines. These two compounds are found in numerous hot and cold beverages including tea, coffee and Coca-Cola. The use of these compounds in human sports

Plate 21 Horses working on gallops on Warren Hill, Newmarket (photograph D. Marlin)

Plate 22 Horse exercising on a treadmill capable of speeds up to 30mph (14 m/sec)

Plate 23 Horse in a swimming pool (photograph D. Marlin)

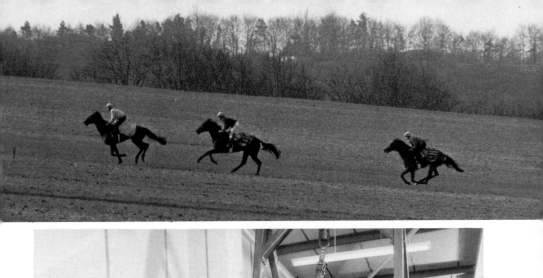

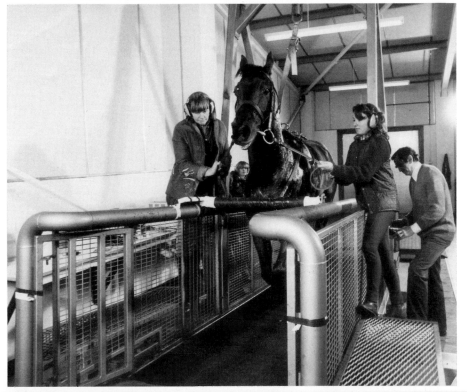

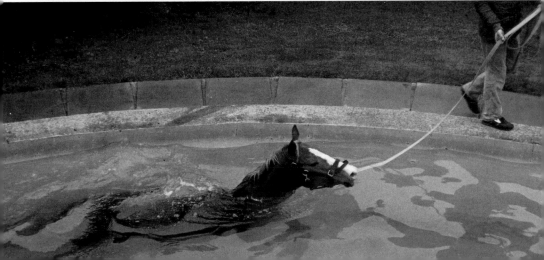

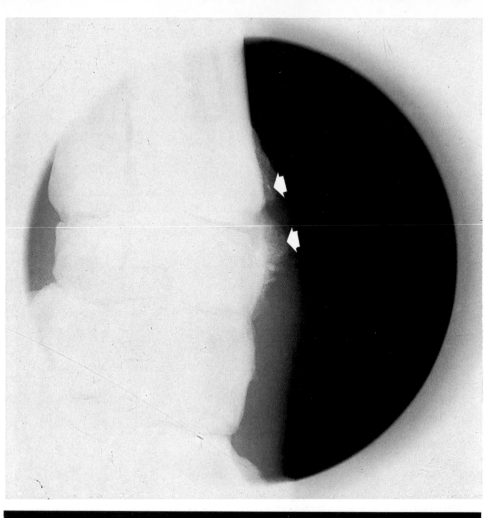

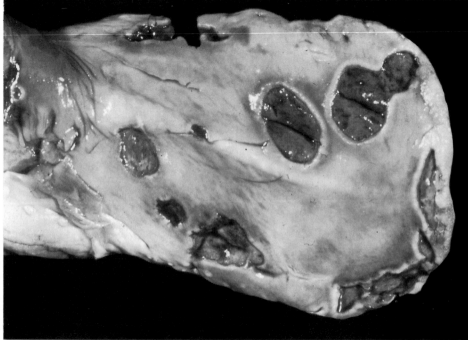

medicine is allowed as long as they are ingested in beverages. However, it is difficult to prove whether the amount detected was from the normal consumption of beverages or if it has been taken as tablets for its stimulant effects. In most racing jurisdictions the use of caffeine and related compounds is illegal. In the UK the strict rules operating have lead to the occasional detection of theobromine in urine samples. In almost all cases, this has been found to be a cause of accidental doping as the theobromine has been traced back to the contamination of a feed supply by this compound. Because of the risk of contamination by feeds containing theobromine used in the preparation of cattle pellets, etc, the larger horse-feed manufacturers have mills that provide pelleted feed solely for racehorse use and guaranteed to be free of theobromine.

Caffeine and the other xanthines exert various effects on the body, as well as those on the central nervous system. The strength of their various effects varies between the compounds, with caffeine having the most potent CNS action. They also have an effect on the heart, lungs, muscle and kidney. Caffeine has also been shown to increase the amount of free fatty acids transported in the blood and therefore recently has found use in marathon runners to prolong their endurance capacity or running speed. In the horse there are two reports on caffeine increasing sprinting speed.

Narcotics   This refers to the group of drugs which are related to morphine and include morphine, heroin, pentazocine and fentanyl (Sublimaze). Drugs derived from the poppy, ie opium, heroin and morphine, have been used since ancient times as the most effective drug for the relief of pain (analgesics). Interestingly, as well as producing analgesia in man, they also cause sedation (narcosis). However, in the horse they produce stimulation reflected in increased locomotory activity. Therefore, as doping agents, their use has been restricted to the horse. For a while it was rumoured that fentanyl was being used extensively in the USA to stimulate horses on the racetrack. This group of drugs and the effects of different doses has been studied extensively by Dr Tobin in Kentucky. Although they have been shown to increase locomotory activity, there is no definitive evidence to indicate whether they actually do improve running speed. At very high doses these drugs produce incoordination.

Plate 24 New bone (indicated by the arrows) formed in a joint after a corticosteroid injection

Plate 25 An example of ulceration that may occur in different parts of the oral cavity and digestive tract following an overdosage of phenylbutazone. Numerous ulcerations on the tongue are shown

Recently, it has been shown that morphine and related compounds exert their effects by acting on specific receptors within the CNS and that a naturally occurring neurotransmitter referred to as enkephalins or endorphins also acts on these receptors. These endorphins are considered to be responsible for lowering the perception of pain and also leading to a tranquil state. It has been suggested that acupuncture exerts its effect by releasing these compounds. Interestingly, a recent report has claimed that the application of a twitch to a horse increases the amount of endorphins, and this explains why painful or worrisome procedures can then be carried out more readily in excitable animals. The normally produced compounds have a very short duration in the body, being destroyed in seconds. Because of these actions, synthetic endorphins are now being manufactured and there have been claims that these have been administered to horses to improve performance or to act as analgesics. Whether these drugs can increase the pain threshold and thus encourage horses to run on, has still to be investigated.

Psychotomimetic drugs (mood enhancers)   These include such compounds as LSD (lysergic acid diethylamide), mescaline and marijuana. Whether they have any effect on athletic performance has not been investigated, although there have been suggestions of marijuana being used in horses.

Miscellaneous   The use of apomorphine, pemoline and strychnine to try to improve performance has been detected in the horse. Strychnine has been detected in a number of attempted and accidental dopings. It is a compound that has been incorporated in a number of stimulant tonic preparations to improve the appetite of horses.

Training aids
Anabolic steroids
The use of anabolic steroids to improve athletic performance is a topic of frequent discussion in newspapers as well as scientific journals. Today, it is probably the most widely used illegal drug in human athletics and is also used by body-builders. The word anabolic means tissue building, as opposed to catabolic which refers to tissue breakdown seen during many disease states. This anabolic activity has been used by athletes in the belief that it promotes the building of muscle mass. This is important because, as described in an earlier chapter, the power that can be developed by a muscle is proportional to its cross-sectional area; therefore any increase in size can be considered beneficial for athletes competing in power events, eg weight-lifting, field events, as well as sprint-

ing. For similar purposes, these compounds have been administered to horses either in the hope of increasing muscle mass for racing or for making horses more presentable at sales.

Anabolic steroids are compounds that are synthesised with chemical structures closely resembling that of the male hormone testosterone which is secreted from the testis. In fact, testosterone is still the most potent anabolic steroid. This also explains why subjects being administered anabolic steroids acquire male characteristics, although attempts have been made to reduce these properties in some compounds. In growing animals it does appear that anabolic steroids do result in increased muscle formation and for this reason have been used in livestock to hasten growth rates. Any increase in muscle mass is due to an increase in the size of individual muscle cells rather than new fibres being produced. It has also been suggested that an increase in muscle size is just due to an increase in their water content. However, in human athletes and possibly the horse, whether any increase in muscle mass in mature animals is due to a direct effect on muscles is controversial. Many argue that the favourable results seen with training are due to the behavioural changes these compounds cause leading to increased aggression and drive. It is thought that these effects permit athletes to train harder, leading to a secondary increase in muscle mass. These compounds may also speed up recovery from minor injuries. In a trial by one of the authors, no favourable effects either on muscle size, composition or on performance were seen when one of these compounds was administered over several months to a group of mature geldings. However, increased aggressive behaviour was seen which persisted for weeks after the cessation of treatment and the detection of the drug in urine samples. In discussion with trainers, differing opinions are held on the beneficial effects of anabolic steroids on performance. Perhaps the fact that geldings can often race as well as stallions also mitigates against their usefulness.

These compounds are also used by veterinarians in treating horses recovering from debilitating conditions as their actions do increase appetite and promote a more efficient utilisation of the feed. Their use in improving red blood cell counts has been suggested, although in the horse there is no strong evidence for this other than a secondary effect through their improving the general well-being of the animal.

Although in man the use of anabolic steroids is now definitely considered illegal, with increasing steps being made to stop its use, the arguments are not as clear in the horse. In man, their use is prevented not only because of the possibility of giving some athletes an unfair advantage but also because of the chance of harmful effects due to prolonged use. In horses, undesirable side-effects, apart from behavioural changes, are not marked. Although reproductive efficiency may be decreased in stallions and mares within a year of cessation of treatment, this is reversible with time. Their use in young growing animals may lead to increases in muscle mass, putting undue strain on immature bones leading to bone problems. To legitamise their use, the argument could be put forward that if it is alright to remove the natural hormone testosterone by gelding animals, why should not a similar compound be given as a partial replacement, at least in geldings.

A number of anabolic steroid preparations are available to the equine practitioner, and some of these only have a very short duration of action while others, because of the manner in which they are given, may persist in the body for over one month. In the UK the main anabolic steroid is a compound referred to as nandrolone, while in the USA it is boldenone. Whether these compounds can be used varies between different racing jurisdictions, often largely depending on whether the specialised methods for detection are available. Naturally, in countries where there is a complete ban on any form of medication, their use is illegal. As a result of the illegality of these compounds both for man and horses, people have resorted to using the natural compound testosterone. However, today the analysts have found methods to distinguish whether the testosterone has been naturally produced or was administered.

Vitamins

These compounds cannot be considered as doping agents and, as far as the authors are aware, their use is not considered illegal. One exception in some places is the intravenous injection of vitamin B_1 (thiamine), as it may cause sedation. It is well known that many human athletes, as well as trainers handling horses, believe that the additions of high amounts of various vitamins may improve performance. Unfortunately, there is little, if any, evidence, largely because no research has been carried out to support this, although there may be a small increase in requirement for some of the B vitamins. However, this should be met by the increased rations given to meet higher energy requirements.

Pangamic acid, often called vitamin B_{15}, is not a true vitamin. It is actually a mixture of a number of compounds which has been claimed to cause an improvement in performance by increasing the oxidative capacity of the body. A number of mechanisms for this have been suggested. However, most well-controlled research in man has not supported this belief, although in a study of racing greyhounds, a significant improvement in times was seen.

Buffers

These are compounds which help to counteract the chemical changes that may cause a shift from the normal neutral pH of the body to either an acid or alkaline state. Normally, in the body there are a number of compounds including proteins, haemoglobin and bicarbonate that aid in this function. As already described, with strenuous short-term exercise, when anaerobic metabolism also occurs to meet the energy needs, lactic acid is produced. The accumulation of this substance results in a progressive decline in pH within muscle cells until a point is reached when processes involved in contraction cannot continue. In order to try to overcome this effect it has been suggested that increasing the buffering capacity of the blood and/or muscle may be useful. For this effect the most commonly tried method is to increase the bicarbonate ion concentration of blood by either giving the compound intravenously or, more commonly, by adding it to the feed. This has been tried in both man and horse, but scientific studies have been carried out to evaluate its effects only with regard to man. Largely due to varying exercise regimes and amounts of bicarbonate given, findings have been equivocal with both some and no improvement in performance occurring. It has been shown that bicarbonate, because it does not enter the cells, only increases the buffering capacity of the blood and this promotes the more rapid passage of lactate from muscle into blood. The use of this compound, because it is a normal nutrient, cannot be considered illegal. However, if any possible effectiveness from this compound is to be gained, fairly high doses have to be used, and these may cause intestinal upsets. Therefore, great care should be taken when adding anything other than low amounts of bicarbonate to the diet. It is also unlikely that continual administration of bicarbonate will have any beneficial effect. Bicarbonate should not be given to horses involved in endurance events during which the blood becomes alkaline rather than acid.

Another substance used to improve buffering capacity is a compound called Tris. This is a buffer used by biochemists, and as it is not a normal nutrient would, in many places, be considered as a doping agent. Tris has the advantage that it enters cells and so also increases their buffering capacity. The effectiveness of this substance in either horse or man has not been thoroughly investigated.

Drugs to restore performance

The wear and tear of training and racing as well as exposure to infectious agents leads to damage to various tissues, which can impair the full responsiveness of the system and loss of performance. In many instances, this damage can be overcome or covered up by the use of various drugs. The pros and cons of whether this should be allowed is considered when the use of anti-inflammatory agents is discussed. The major drugs in this category may be classed as follows:

1 Drugs to relieve pain:

    a) Anti-inflammatory agents of both the non-steroidal (eg phenylbutazone) and corticosteroid (eg cortisone) types. These are used to alleviate inflammations resulting from injury and disease, with their most common use being to treat lameness.
    b) Local anaesthetics. These are most frequently used to inject painful joints.

2 Drugs to overcome respiratory problems that hinder the high air-flows and gas exchanges necessary at high speeds.

Pain and the athletic horse
It has been suggested that 'pain is an occupational hazard in sports'. We have no way of knowing whether this is true of equine sports in the same way as it is claimed to be in human sports, but there are certainly times when the athletic horse will feel pain during a competition. Basically, this pain occurs in three types of situation. First, the horse may have a long-standing chronic veterinary problem, eg an arthritis, which is aggravated by exercise but which does not prevent the horse from exercising. Secondly, the horse may injure itself during a competition. Thirdly, the horse may feel pain due to muscle fatigue, etc. This type of pain would normally pass off, of course, when the horse has recuperated after exercise. The causes of the pain associated with fatigue have been discussed in an earlier chapter.

    Over the ages, man has made a number of attempts to counteract the effects of pain in his horses in order to prolong their working life or to improve their performance. Two types of drugs can now be employed to this end: anti-inflammatory drugs and pain-killers. In some cases, one drug, such as phenylbutazone, will have both effects. Each of these drugs will be discussed in turn.

Inflammation and the corticosteroids
The corticosteroids were one of the first anti-inflammatory drugs to be used. Initially, a natural compound, cortisol, was used but nowadays synthetic corticosteroids are used. In addition to its effect on inflammation, cortisol causes the body to retain sodium and water which would otherwise be eliminated via the kidneys. The pharmaceutical industry has discovered newer and newer variations on the cortisone theme which have ever-increasing anti-inflammatory action but cause less and less sodium retention (Table 28). Although we now know a great

deal about how to make new corticosteroids, we still do not know exactly how they work. It is thought that they are taken into the nucleus of cells and cause them to alter the proteins which are made by that cell. They have the same effects whether they are injected locally into a precise area, such as a joint, or are administered to the horse as a whole.

Table 28   Relative effects of natural and synthetic corticosteroids

Drug		Amount of sodium retention	Anti-inflammatory action
Natural	Cortisol	1	1
Synthetic	Prednisolone	0.8	4
	Dexamethasone	0	25
	Flumethasone	0	700

Inflamation is recognised by the affected area becoming hot, red (although in horses this may not be very evident) and swollen. Corticosteroids reduce all these effects. They are not without their problems, however. The main problem is that they do nothing at all about the root cause of the trouble. For example, a horse with sweet-itch will rub its mane and tail areas red raw. If we inject the horse with corticosteroids, it will stop rubbing and the skin will start to heal. When the injection wears off, however, all the symptoms will come back because we have done nothing to prevent the fly bites which are at the root cause of the situation. If, on the other hand, the horse is kept in a fly-proof stable twenty-four hours a day, then the symptoms will disappear without the need for any drugs because the causal factor has been removed. In the athletic horse, it was soon realised that when a horse's joints started to show symptoms of wear and tear, and arthritis of varying kinds appeared, then an injection of corticosteroid directly into the affected joint could bring about a miraculous improvement. Within a short time the horse would use the joint almost normally. The problem was that the root cause, whether excessive work, old age, etc, was not being relieved. A number of such horses would suddenly go very lame at a later date because the joint tissues had literally collapsed. When this happens, the joint is beyond any veterinary help. It follows that great care must be taken in selecting horses for intra-articular injection of corticosteroids, and any owner who allows his horse to be injected must realise the danger of possible future damage (Plate 24).

If we seem to be concentrating on the adverse effects of corticosteroids, this is because when an owner is faced with severely decreased athletic performance in his horse, all too often the pressure to take the short-term gain overshadows the long-term consequences. Even in the short term, however, there may be a post-injection inflammatory reaction in the joint after intra-articular injection of a corticosteroid. Further, unless great care has been taken to ensure that the injection was given under sterile conditions, the joint may develop a septic arthritis. This is because corticosteroids not only reduce the bad effects of inflammation, they also reduce the good effects. As a result, the joint (or the whole body if the drug is administered parenterally) has a much reduced resistance to infection. In the long term, in addition to the kind of joint collapse which has already been mentioned, long-acting corticosteroids may cause new bone to be formed around the joint.

The corticosteroids have a number of effects on the horse's body as a whole, especially if they are given over any length of time. As happens in man, they can cause a feeling of well-being. This has, on occasions, led to their being abused to dope a horse and encourage it to perform better. Another of the effects within the body is to reduce the amount of adrenocorticotrophic hormone (ACTH) which is released from the anterior pituitary gland. This occurs because ACTH is normally released whenever the horse is stressed and needs more natural corticosteroid. With large amounts of artificial corticosteroid present, the ACTH mechanism becomes 'rusty'. When the injection wears off, however, it may be some time before the ACTH release reaches normal levels. During this time the horse may be unthrifty, dull and depressed. Anyone buying a horse which has been performing well prior to purchase, but which does not do well after purchase, and shows any of these symptoms, may well suspect that they are now paying the price for drug-induced performance.

The corticosteroids do have one advantage over some of the other drugs which are used to reduce inflammation. They are not pain-killers as such. If a horse is in less pain on corticosteroids, then this is because the drug has actually reduced the inflammation which is causing the pain. With some other drugs, as we shall see, the horse may appear to be improving, but only because a general pain-killing effect is masking the fact that there has been no improvement in the underlying condition.

The use of non-steroidal drugs to counteract inflammation
The most commonly used group of drugs in the athletic horse is probably the non-steroidal anti-inflammatory agents (NSAIDs). As their name implies, none of these drugs have the steroidal chemical structure of cortisol. They do, however, all have a similar mode of action and some common chemical features. At the present time, the NSAIDs which are most commonly used in the horse are phenylbutazone (often referred to as 'bute'), meclofenamic acid, naproxen and flunixin. As each new drug has

come onto the market, it has been hailed as being more effective than its predecessors. It has also almost invariably been more expensive than its predecessors. In the UK, for example, a dose of naproxen will now cost around twenty times as much as a dose of phenylbutazone for the same horse. One of the practical results of this is that it puts great pressure on people to use the older, but potentially more toxic drugs, such as phenyl-butazone. At the same time, the veterinary surgeon is much more likely to overprescribe the cheaper drug, and so horse owners are much more likely to acquire a stock of the drug which they can use to medicate that horse, or another one with a completely different problem, without seek-ing professional advice.

NSAIDs are all acidic chemicals, and this has a great bearing on their use. As a result of this low acidity, they have very low solubility in water. In an attempt to counteract this, they are often made up as the sodium salt, and this also helps them to be absorbed better when they are given by mouth. The low acidity does have the advantage that it helps the drug to accumulate in inflamed areas of the horse's body. Another important chemical property is that, once they get into the body, a high proportion of the drug becomes bound together with pro-teins in the blood plasma. With meclofenamic acid or naproxen, for example, over 99 per cent of the drug which is administered will become bound to proteins in this way. It is, however, the free drug, which is not bound to protein, which is active. So, relatively large amounts of the drug must be given in order to achieve sufficient levels of the free drug to be clinically active. A further complication is that if another drug which becomes bound to proteins is given at the same time as a NSAID, then both drugs will have less protein-bound drug than normal, and so more active drug than normal. One practical implication of this is that both warfarin (which is used to treat navicular disease) and phenylbutazone (which is used as a painkiller in navicular disease) become protein bound. If both are given together, the horse may, in fact, be receiving a dangerous dose of active warfarin.

To understand how these drugs work, it is necessary to look first at some of the activity which takes place in inflamed areas of the body. During the inflammatory process, a substance called arachidonic acid is converted into various prostaglandins, etc. These prostaglandins are the chemicals which actually cause the symptoms of heat, swelling, pain, etc. They also markedly increase the sensitivity of pain receptors in inflamed areas to the agents which cause pain. The change from arachidonic acid to prostaglandin needs an enzyme, or catalyst, to be present before it can take place, and this enzyme is called cyclo-oxygenase. The NSAID drugs appear to act by 'neutralising' the cyclo-oxygenase. Without the enzyme, no prostaglandins can be formed, and the symptoms of inflammation will disappear once any existing prostaglandins have been used up.

Because of the various regulations governing the use of drugs which are given to horses competing in various spheres, it is important to understand how the drugs are eliminated from the horse's body. Most of the NSAIDs will eventually be broken down in the horse's liver to completely inactive substances. These inactive substances, or metabolites, are then eliminated from the body via the urine or bile. There are a couple of practical points which follow from this. First, very little of these drugs is eliminated via the saliva, so taking saliva samples from horses is not an accurate way of telling whether they have been given one of these drugs. Secondly, because urine and bile are the ultimate destination of these drugs, it is usually possible to detect them or their metabolites for a much longer period in urine than it is in blood. The irony of this is that, from time to time, proposals from various official bodies to take blood samples for dope testing have been strenuously opposed by owners and riders, even though such testing would, in some cases, be much less sensitive than the existing urine testing and so would make detection of the drugs less certain. Yet these same people will often complain that modern advances in drug detection have gone too far because it is now possible to pick up minute traces of drugs which have no clinical significance. This brings us to the third point. Because of the high protein-binding properties of the NSAIDs, it is probable that they are still present in tissues (even in sufficient concentrations to have some effect) for some time after they can be detected in blood, etc. This is why horses which are chronically lame, for instance, will remain improved for three or four days after the last dose of a NSAID.

The 'Bute' controversy

Phenylbutazone was the first of the modern NSAIDs to be used in horses. Although it has been used for many years, it is only comparatively recently that we have found out much about its effect. It is almost as if people were initially so relieved to find a drug which was so effective at reducing inflammation and at making horses which were lame with navicular disease, for example, sound again, that they did not bother to research any further into the drug. Phenylbutazone is most commonly given by mouth. This raises a problem because the chemical itself is very bitter to the taste. This is overcome by coating the granules of the drug with a tasteless preparation which masks the taste. Despite this, there are some horses which can detect phenylbutazone in concentrations almost as small as the analytical chemist, and such horses will not touch medicated feed. To overcome this problem, the drug is now available in a paste formulation which can be squirted into the horse's mouth.

The timing of phenylbutazone administration by mouth can be very important. If it is given on an empty stomach, which in practical terms usually means that it is given first thing in the morning, then more of the drug is absorbed than if it is given later in the day when the stomach is full (Fig 42). This is because the more food there is in the stomach, the slower the stomach will empty itself. Phenylbutazone is absorbed in the small intestine, so the slower the stomach empties, the longer it will be before the drug reaches the small intestine. In the case of ponies, it would appear that they have a relatively small stomach compared with horses. The stomach emptying time is therefore relatively short, and they absorb proportionally more of the drug compared with horses. This can cause problems, as we will discuss later.

Phenylbutazone can also be given by intravenous injection (although not by intramuscular injection because it is too irritant when given by this route). This has the advantage that you remove the uncertainties

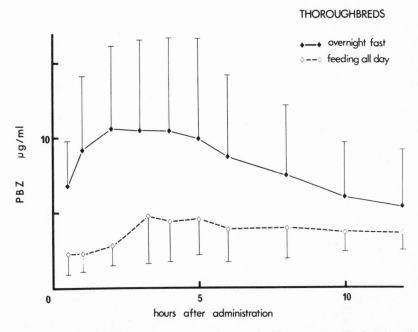

THOROUGHBREDS

●——● overnight fast
◇--◇ feeding all day

Fig 42 Concentration of phenylbutazone in the plasma following the oral administration of approximately 2gm of the drug. Note the much lower amounts when the drug is given on a full stomach, although not shown here, levels may increase in the next 14 hours due to delayed absorption. The vertical lines from each point indicate the large variability that occurs between animals

associated with giving it by mouth. This can be especially important if an attempt is being made to keep a horse on the drug while still keeping blood levels below an officially permissible limit. At the present time, for instance, FEI (the International Equestrian Federation) allow blood levels of no more than 5μg phenylbutazone and oxyphenbutazone per ml of blood in horses competing in their official competitions. Giving the drug intravenously also means that it will be acting within the horse's body two or three hours earlier than if it was given by mouth. The actual size of the dose which is given determines, in the case of phenylbutazone, how long the drug will last in the body. If a horse is given, for example, 4.4mg/kg of phenylbutazone then its half life (which is the time taken for half the drug to be eliminated) will be 3½ hours. If the dose were to be increased to 8.8mg/kg, then the half life of the drug would be almost doubled to 6 hours.

Phenylbutazone had been used in horses for about thirty years before any real effort was made to see whether there were any toxicity problems with the drug, despite the fact that several problems were known to occur in man. In the UK, the drug is no longer available for general prescription in man, and it can only be prescribed by a hospital specialist for certain specific conditions. Used at the recommended dose levels (and these have been amended in recent years as a result of the toxicity research), phenylbutazone causes few apparent problems in horses, even after prolonged administration. In ponies, however, giving it at doses only slightly above normal for up to a week can cause serious problems and even death. What happens is that the drug affects the lining of the intestines in such a way that they allow proteins to leak out into the intestinal contents and be eliminated from the body. In time, large ulcers develop, especially in the large intestine and also on the tongue (Plate 25). It is the loss of protein which can cause oedema, or the accumulation of tissue fluid, to occur and which is responsible for the fatalities. Although horses, as has been mentioned, appear much less susceptible to these problems than ponies, changes in the blood protein levels do occur in horses and occasional blood checks should be carried out on any horses receiving phenylbutazone for long periods.

Phenylbutazone is broken down in the horse's liver ready for its 'disposal'. One unusual feature of the drug compared with the other NSAIDs is that about 10 per cent of it is broken down into a metabolite called oxyphenbutazone, and this is itself clinically active. The practical effect of this is that whenever an official body wishes to limit the use of phenylbutazone, they also have to link this with restrictions on the use of oxyphenbutazone because otherwise there would be a strong temptation for horse owners to switch to using the other metabolite.

Choosing which NSAID to use

Because of prolonged experienced with its use, and its low cost, phenyl-butazone has tended to become the standard first choice drug to treat many inflammatory conditions of the muscles, bones, etc. The NSAIDs are, however, all slightly different and each has its strengths and weaknesses. In practice, phenylbutazone is most effective in relieving bony conditions such as chronic arthritis of varying kinds. It is less effective at treating the myositis, or muscle inflammation, which occurs in horses with azoturia. In this situation, naproxen is a much more effective drug. Naproxen has been shown to be effective in improving over 90 per cent of horses with clinical myositis. The drug is available as a powder, which is not bitter to the taste and so is accepted relatively easily by horses.

An interesting experiment has been carried out where yearling quarterhorse colts in training were given either low doses of naproxen every day or nothing except normal treatment for any problems which occurred. The treated horses lost significantly fewer days from training (3 per cent compared with 13 per cent). They also raced more often and had up to thirty times fewer musculoskeletal problems than the other group. This raises the question of whether such research shows that anti-inflammatory drugs could be given beneficially to all young horses in training. One would really want to look at the long-term results in the treated horses, and also compare X-rays of their limbs with those of untreated horses, before making such a revolutionary suggestion.

Naproxen is rapidly broken down in the horse's body, so much so that it has to be given twice a day in order to keep blood levels high enough to be effective. This lack of accumulation of the drug results in a very low toxicity. In contrast to the situation with phenylbutazone, as much as three times the recommended dose has been given for six weeks without any side-effects appearing.

Like naproxen, meclofenamic acid can only be given to horses by mouth. It is, however, quite palatable and so this presents few problems. It is unusual because, although plasma levels of the drug rise to a peak within 4 hours of the initial dose, the clinical effect may not be seen for 36-96 hours after dosing. Despite this delay, the plasma levels decline over 24 hours, and daily dosage is necessary. The drug is claimed to be up to twelve times as potent as phenylbutazone in reducing inflammation. This activity may rise from an ability to prevent certain inflammatory cells, such as monocytes, from invading inflamed areas and so preventing them from releasing prostaglandins, etc. Meclofenamic acid may be particularly effective in relieving laminitis.

The most recent NSAID on the horse scene in the UK has been fluni-xin. This can be given by injection (either intravenously or intramuscularly), or orally. The drug has a very short half life in the horse's plasma after intravenous injection, although its clinical effect will last for up to thirty hours.

Unusually among the NSAIDs, flunixin has been found to be very effective at reducing the pain associated with colic in the horse. As, however, this relief can occur within literally minutes of the injection, there is some uncertainty as to how this effect is achieved. Peak activity in musculoskeletal inflammation is not seen until 12-16 hours after initial dosing.

As already mentioned, the use of NSAIDs is allowed in certain racing jurisdictions, although the period when they can be administered prior to racing does vary. Strong arguments have been put by both those in favour of permitting the use of the drugs and those against, and some of these are summarised below.

1 Arguments against:

1 People consider any kind of treatment unfair and artificial.
2 Allowing even limited use of certain drugs leads to difficulties in controlling their correct use.
3 By masking pain, the use of drugs such as NSAIDs may lead to abnormal requests on the horse's physical capabilities.
4 Giving NSAIDs to unsound animals in order to compete may result in the existing physical problem getting worse.
5 Medication may result in horses breaking down during competition, thereby risking further injury to both horse and rider.
6 Horses with inherent conformation defects may be able to overcome them by the use of drugs and this may lead to the selection of faulty conformation for breeding purposes.

2 Arguments in favour:

1 These drugs cannot be considered as stimulants as they are unlikely to effect a horse's optimal performance. The drugs do, however, by their pain-killing and anti-inflammatory effects, improve performance towards normal by allowing normal functioning of joints, etc. For example, stride length will be greater while on NSAIDs than off them if there are joint problems.
2 In the USA it is argued that there is a lack of sound horses to fill all the races being held throughout the country, and therefore a loss of betting revenue would follow their banning. Frequent racing of each individual horse is necessary to even start to recover the cost of racehorse ownership.
3 Horses aimed at FEI events require long and vigorous training which must put a strain on the horse and cause some unsoundness. The banning of such drugs must lead to fewer horses lasting the course and reaching the top of their field.
4 The use of neurectomy (cutting the nerves which supply the horse's foot) is a much worse alternative treatment for chronic lameness.

5 Few horses entering FEI competitions are used for breeding, therefore the use of drugs would not effect the conformation, etc of blood-lines.
6 There is claimed to be no evidence of NSAIDs causing undesirable side-effects in competing horses.
7 Banning all of these drugs means that they cannot be used either to treat or prevent minor traumatic injuries occurring during competitions which may last several days.
8 NSAIDs other than phenylbutazone are allowed to be used by human athletes in Olympic competitions.

During the past two or three years there has been a marked change in people's attitudes to even the use of these drugs in competing horses. The work on the toxicity of phenylbutazone, which has already been mentioned, appeared to have a catalytic effect in making people on the fringes of the horse world question the morality of allowing the use of such drugs on a long-term basis to cope with chronic problems. At the same time, of course, there has been a general interest in 'animal rights', often among people who are not involved at all in the general care of horses, let alone involved in competitions. The result has been that a few countries have passed legislation specifically banning the use of all drugs in horses involved in such competitions. This is civil legislation, not merely 'in house' rules agreed between those involved with the sport. Even the USA, where phenylbutazone was once allowed in horse-racing in most states, is changing its attitude. A number of states have now banned the use of such drugs, and a few years ago federal legislation was even under consideration to extend this ban over the whole of the union. Time will tell what the effect of these bans will be both on the individual horses affected and on the competition world as a whole.

Local anaesthetics and nerve blocks
The anti-inflammatory drugs which might be used to restore a horse's well-being after the wear and tear of performance are generally administered to the whole animal and remove some of the naturally produced substances that are responsible for the signs of inflammation (including pain). Where the pain can be localised to a specific joint or tendon, a more local approach can be used. This involves 'blocking' the nerve that transmits the sensation of pain from the region. To do this a local anaesthetic is injected around the nerve, or into the joint to diffuse to the nerve endings in the joint capsule. If the site of pain is numbed, the animal can run sound, and for this reason local anaesthesia has been used in race and competition horses. Besides being banned by most regulatory bodies, such a practice poses a risk both to horse and rider. This is because the lack of pain causes the horse to perform normally and

therefore risks damage which could be extremely serious, eg the complete rupture of a tendon. Occasionally, the local anaesthetic can also escape into the blood and enter the brain, causing marked excitement. There are a number of local anaesthetics available, including procaine, lignocaine and benzocaine. They all have a short duration of action with their effects wearing off within a couple of hours. They are all easily detected in routine dope tests.

In some cases the nerve is physically cut by surgery in order to give long-lasting pain relief. It is long lasting rather than permanent because in many cases sensation will return after two or three years. Unlike the local anaesthetics, this practice cannot be detected with any degree of certainty. Its principal use has been in alleviating the symptoms of navicular disease in order to allow the horse to continue to perform. The possible consequences of such long-lasting loss of sensation are obvious, including the fact that infections and injuries can establish themselves in the foot without anyone being the wiser.

Respiratory drugs
As already outlined in the chapter describing the respiratory system, respiratory performance increases markedly with exercise and there are a number of clinical conditions which can impair performance. In older animals the condition of chronic obstructive pulmonary disease (heaves) can occur. Present opinion is that this is an allergic condition and therefore, not surprisingly, it has been found that drugs that are used in human asthmatics can alleviate or overcome these conditions to restore normal respiratory function. However, these are usually only effective in the early stages of the disease, as with time irreversible damage occurs. Essentially, two types of drug are used. One is a compound called sodium cromoglycate (Cromovet[R]) which is the same as Intal used in man. This prevents cells releasing compounds that cause constriction of smaller airways when exposed to allergens. This compound is therefore a prophylactic (preventive agent) and has no effect once the allergen exerts itself. The other group of agents are bronchodilators, and, as their name implies, they overcome the constriction of the airways. The most important drugs are those that closely resemble adrenalin but only exert some of this compound's effects. These compounds include salbutamol and terbutaline, both extensively employed in human asthmatics. In addition, there is a drug available only to veterinarians called clenbuterol (Ventipulmin). This is an extremely potent compound and therefore requires only very small doses to be given, making detection difficult, although not impossible. There is evidence that these drugs have been used illegally to try to improve perfor-

mance. In the normal animal not suffering from constricted airways the drug has no favourable effect.

Side-effects from these drugs can be seen especially if given in slightly higher doses than recommended for therapeutic use. These effects are related to their adrenalin actions, resulting in muscle tremor, sweating and an increased heart rate.

Exercise-induced pulmonary haemorrhage (EIPH) has now been shown to be of common occurrence in racehorses, although epistaxis (ie bleeding) is less frequent. For a number of years it has been thought that the drug frusemide (Lasix^R) could either completely or partially prevent bleeding and improve performance. It has therefore found widespread use on the racetracks in North America in both Standardbred and Thoroughbred racing, being administered pre-race. Unfortunately, most of the research on its effectiveness has not borne out this belief, held not only by trainers but also by track veterinary surgeons. However, a recent study has indicated that the degree of EIPH may be reduced by Lasix. If it works, how it may have a beneficial effect is largely unknown, although several mechanisms have been suggested. Normally, Lasix is used as a diuretic, ie a drug that increases fluid removal by the kidneys. It is potent in this action, exerting its effect within minutes of its administration and causing up to a fifty-fold increase in the amount of urine voided. Today, the use of this drug pre-race is permitted medication in a number of states in the USA.

Epilogue: The Future

The up-to-date scientific knowledge which we have been discussing in this book opens up all sorts of exciting possibilities for the individual horse owner and trainer who is interested in achieving the most from the athletic horse. It is, however, only the beginning. There is so much that we still do not know about how the horse 'works', and so much more scope for improving the way we approach the whole concept of exercise in the horse world.

It has often been pointed out that, despite intensive breeding programmes involving horses of ever-increasing values, the Thoroughbred horse is no better at racing now than it was several decades ago. It is certainly true that the speed of the racehorse has improved only slightly, if at all, and many racing records are of very long standing. There are several factors which might be responsible for this apparent lack of progress besides failure to improve the breed.

1   In some ways, Thoroughbred breeding reached its peak at the turn of the century. Since that time stud books have been under very strict control, and so breeders have, to all intents and purposes, been working within a closed genetic pool. They can cross one 'family' with another, but they cannot bring in a completely new family from outside to introduce hybrid vigour. Contrast this situation with the human athletic world, where records are continually tumbling, but where modern communications have led to so much intermingling of races and colours.

2   Some of the human records which have fallen have done so because the athlete has been prepared to train hard and go through the pain barrier. We cannot expect to be able to train horses to this level – we cannot motivate them to fulfil our human ambitions.

3   In European racing especially, there is no extra prize money available if a horse does beat a record. Winning on the day is the sole aim, and so tactics are more important than sheer performance. It might be that the promoters of racing in the USA are more adventurous in this field. Certainly, race times are a vital part of racing in that country, helping in the comparison of different horses which might not have many opportunities to race against each other because of the great distances involved.

4   Improvements have been made in track surfaces, etc, which may have increased overall performance and decreased the risk of tendon 'break-downs', but which have lessened the gap between the best and the less able horse.

5   In Europe, there is now a far greater tendency to water courses. 'Good' going may suit more horses than 'fast' going, but it does not produce such fast speeds.

6   The high prices which successful horses can now command since they became a commodity to be traded like gold or silver have resulted in a greater temptation to remove a successful horse from the track and send it to stud.

It would be wrong to be too gloomy about the present situation. Modern training methods give the horse a chance to achieve its genetic potential, and the resulting fitness enables it to work at this maximum potential for longer periods. We must also remember that the factors limiting physical performance vary according to both the nature of the exercise and the environment in which it is being carried out. Our race-tracks have changed little over the years. The facilities for the racegoers are continually being improved, but little research is carried out with a view to improving things for the horses, ie reducing the strains placed upon the horse at speed. In the fields of showjumping and cross-country, things have changed markedly. The courses are very much stiffer than they used to be, so little improvement can be expected. If we want to see the same advances in equine performances as are taking place in human athletics, then we may need to adopt the same team approach that they do. This would mean that every serious competition yard would have ready access to the following specialists: veterinary surgeon; exercise physiologist; farrier; nutritionist; biomechanics expert; radiologist; physiotherapist. Some racing trainers are starting to think this way already.

As we have constantly stressed, there is still much we would like to know. Very little research has yet been carried out on the effects of exercise on bones and tendons. This is partly because we do not have a biopsy technique to enable us to take samples of the bones and tendons before, during, and after exercise. The great advance in our knowledge of muscles which has followed the introduction of the percutaneous needle biopsy technique which has already been described shows what can be achieved. Nor can we catch hold of the coat tails of human research in these fields because man does not have the long tendons which the horse has, and the forces on his tendons are very much less.

There is still much we would like to know about how a horse moves.

259

We have progressed a long way from the early photographic solution to the question of whether a horse was ever completely suspended in air or not, but we still cannot say what is significant in the way a horse moves and what is not. Horses used on treadmills as described earlier appear less able to cope with conformational 'defects' than when they perform normally. It may be that this is due to the relatively unyielding nature of the surface over which they move compared with natural surfaces such as grass. Certainly, we do not understand the effects of wear and tear on normal joints, let alone slightly abnormal ones. At one time in the Sixties it was claimed that all joint movement, normal or otherwise, could be understood in a relatively simple mathematical way. We now see that as the 'innocence of youth' in a very complex field.

The horse world generally has seen an expansion in the interest in physiotherapy for horses. Here again, a technique as widely used as faradism lacks any really detailed knowledge as to what it is doing and how it is doing it. The muscle masses which propel the horse are so much greater than those in human athletes, and there is, as yet, no proof that such techniques can penetrate to significant depths. It may be that in the future we will see some much needed research into electromyography, looking at the electrical changes which take place in muscles during exercise and at how the nerves control muscle activities. You will notice that there is not a chapter in this book dealing specifically with the nervous system, even though the athletic horse could obviously not perform without an efficient nervous control. The reason for this apparent omission is that we do not yet have much precise information on the horse's nervous system, and it may be inaccurate to assume merely that the horse works in exactly the same way as do laboratory animals or human beings.

The ever-increasing costs of keeping horses will probably ensure that there will be research into horse nutrition in the future. At present, the horse world spends far too much money on so-called feed supplements, and far too little attention to the basic provision of the correct energy and protein levels for the particular work which an individual horse is undertaking. Such incentives for research in the academic world will, however, have to be balanced by the fact that the horse-feed industry is becoming more and more competitive. Already in the UK some of the larger feed companies are having to look very hard at any research budgets because they are competing in the market place with small companies which spend nothing at all on research.

Economics will also play a large part in determining what, if any, new drugs come on to the equine market over the next decade. Although the value of individual horses can be very high, both in economic and in sentimental terms, the fact remains that there are relatively few horses in the world compared with the numbers of cattle or of human beings. The potential market for an equine drug is relatively small. At the same time, the costs of registering such a drug are the same as for one having a much larger potential market. Consumer protection legislation increases in most countries of the world every year, for very commendable reasons. The bureaucracy involved in drug registration can add two years to the time between discovery of a drug and its appearance on the veterinary market.

In the past, a number of drugs became accepted in the equine world via the back door. They were drugs which had been developed for use in human beings, and veterinary surgeons treating horses with similar disease problems tried them and found them useful. As the amounts of these drugs used in the horse increased, manufacturers started to take notice and considered bringing out a veterinary formulation. Nowadays, the temptation is for drug companies to positively discourage any veterinary interest in their human drugs. They fulfil the minimum testing for side-effects required by the registration authorities, but they do not want to run the risk of a side-effect turning up in a horse which might involve them in 'unnecessary' problems with the registration authorities and might even jeopardise their whole human market.

Future legislation is unlikely ever to make registration of drugs easier, and may sometimes have quite unexpected results. For example, moves at present underway in the UK to make the horse an 'agricultural animal' would mean that it would also be considered a meat animal and so all drugs used in the horse would have to specify withdrawal times before the meat would be fit for human consumption.

It would be wrong to finish on such a pessimistic note. The whole aim of the book is to provide horse trainers, whether they look after one horse or one hundred, with a scientific basis for the training methods they use. Where our new knowledge contradicts their established methods, it is to be hoped that they will be able to develop new methods that have a more rational basis. We must at all times remember that the horse is a very specialised animal. It has evolved over thousands of years to gallop at speed (ideally faster than the predators which were pursuing it). By understanding more perfectly how it does so, we can avoid placing undue demands on our horses. They, in their turn, will repay us by the pleasure which so many people get from admiring the athletic horse.

Acknowledgements

The authors are grateful to colleagues at the Animal Health Trust, Newmarket for the many helpful comments. An expert on the topic of each chapter kindly read that chapter. Special thanks go to Professor A. Littlejohn for assistance on the chapter on the respiratory system and Drs D. Leach, D. Wilson, R. Harris and M. Moss, and Miss P. Harris for their constructive comments. Dr J. Mumford provided current information on viral vaccination programmes. However, at the end of the day all mistakes and omissions are the responsibility of the authors. Many of the studies referred to in the text were carried out by one of the authors (DHS) and colleagues. Such studies would not have been possible without financial support from the Horserace Betting Levy Board and the Animal Health Trust. Without the availability of horses for the investigation of new ideas, much of the information presented would not have been possible, and therefore DHS is extremely grateful to those who have expertly cared for his own group of horses. In addition, a number of Thoroughbred trainers, especially C. Brittain, M. Stoute and Sir M. Prescott have allowed ready access to their valuable animals. Without such cooperation the practical application of new approaches could not have been undertaken. DHS is extremely grateful to Mrs Paula Diver for assistance in the typing of the manuscript, whilst CJV is indebted to his wife Susan's patience during the hours spent with his Macintosh computer in writing this book.

Index

INDEX